Environmental Enrichment

for Captive Animals

The Universities Federation for Animal Welfare

UFAW, founded in 1926, is an internationally recognised, independent, scientific and educational animal welfare charity concerned with promoting high standards of welfare for farm, companion, laboratory and captive wild animals, and for those animals with which we interact in the wild. It works to improve animals' lives by:

- Promoting and supporting developments in science and technology that underpin advances in animal welfare

- Promoting education in animal care and welfare

- Providing information, organising meetings, and publishing books, videos, articles, technical reports and the journal *Animal Welfare*

- Providing expert advice to government departments and other bodies and helping to draft and amend laws and guidelines

- Enlisting the energies of animal keepers, scientists, veterinarians, lawyers and others who care about animals

'Improvements in the care of animals are not now likely to come of their own accord, merely by wishing them: there must be research ... and it is in sponsoring research of this kind, and making its results widely known, that UFAW performs one of its most valuable services.'

Sir Peter Medawar CBE FRS, 8th May 1957
Nobel Laureate (1960), Chaiman of the UFAW Scientific Advisory Committee (1951–1962)

For further information about UFAW and about how you can help to promote and support its work, please contact us at the address below.

Universities Federation for Animal Welfare
The Old School, Brewhouse Hill, Wheathampstead, Herts AL4 8AN, UK
Tel: 01582 831818 Fax: 01582 831414 Website: www.ufaw.org.uk

Environmental Enrichment for Captive Animals

Robert J. Young

Series editors:
James K. Kirkwood, Robert C. Hubrecht and Elizabeth A. Roberts

Blackwell Science Ltd, a Blackwell Publishing company
Editorial Offices:
Blackwell Science Ltd, 9600 Garsington Road, Oxford OX4 2DQ, UK
Tel: +44 (0) 1865 776868
Blackwell Publishing Professional, 2121 State Avenue, Ames, Iowa, 50014-8300, USA
Tel: +1 515 292 0140
Blackwell Science Asia Pty Ltd, 550 Swanston Street, Carlton, Victoria 3053, Australia
Tel: +61 (0)3 8359 1011

First published 2003 by Blackwell Science Ltd

7 2010

ISBN: 978-0-6320-6407-6

Library of Congress Cataloging-in-Publication Data
Young, Robert John, 1966–
    Environmental enrichment for captive animals / Robert John Young.
      p. cm.
    Includes bibliographical references (p.).
    I SBN: 978-0-6320-6407-6 (pbk.)
       1. Environmental enrichment (Animal culture).   2. Animal welfare.
       3. Captive wild animals.   4. Domestic animals.   I. Title.

    HV4737.Y68   2003
    636.08′32–dc21

                                                        2002155056

A catalogue record for this title is available from the British Library

Set in 10/12.5 pt Sabon
by SNP Best-set Typesetter Ltd., Hong Kong
Printed and bound in Malaysia by Vivar Printing Sdn Bhd.

For further information on
Blackwell Publishing, visit our website:
www.blackwellpublishing.com

Contents

Preface

This book is born out of my research and practical experience of environmental enrichment. I have tried to write a book that is scientifically rigorous but also practical. First and foremost, I believe that anyone involved in environmental enrichment needs a good basic understanding of animal welfare and the scientific evidence that environmental enrichment does indeed improve animal welfare. However, I did not wish to write a solely theoretical book as these already exist (Shepherdson *et al.*, 1998) and I feel that such theorising is more appropriately published in peer-review journals. The other danger is to go too far the other way and write a practical implementation book, but these also already exist (Field, 1998). Instead, I have opted for the rather more perilous middle path – the hybrid. Really in order to meet the needs of my intended audience. This book is designed for the reader who wishes not only to implement environmental enrichment but also to understand how it actually improves animal welfare. The book is not aimed at the academic researcher in animal welfare, nor is it for those who only want a list of enrichment ideas for the species in their care. The book is not example driven but goal and strategy driven, because there are simply too many species on this planet to cover, more than 4000 mammal species alone.

The content of the book reflects the need for scientific knowledge and practical application of this knowledge. I have based the chapters on those subjects about which I am most frequently questioned either in academic or practical circles. For example, Chapter 12 on 'Designing and Analysing Enrichment Studies' results from the large number of people who have requested this information, principally zoo biologists and university students.

I have also tried to convey much of my own personal experience, both academic and in implementing environmental enrichment. On too many occasions I have visited institutions where people have tried to convey the right scientific and practical information about environmental enrichment but without either sufficient interpersonal skills or enough understanding of the situation to do so effectively. To be serious about the application of environmental enrichment or any animal welfare related subject, you must also be serious about human psychology. It is only by understanding the people who work with animals that environmental enrichment can be successfully implemented. One can have the best academic mind about the subject and the best practical skills for implementation, and yet these will count for nothing without the ability to understand, communicate with, learn from and educate those working with animals.

I regard this as a 'how to' book – by their nature such books are filled with instructions. This book has its fair share of these instructions, but also includes a significant amount on basic principles. Finally, I have tried to write in an accessible style and have in many places given full explanations of concepts rather than simply referring the reader to other literature. This being said, I have often summarised concepts for the sake of brevity, and therefore I highly recommend that, whenever possible the interested reader uses this book in conjunction with the primary sources of information.

This book should not be judged on its sales or academic reviews but by how it is used by the people who read it. My hope is that it may help the more academically minded person produce environmental enrichment that is not only scientifically valid but, importantly, practical. Conversely, I hope that this book will enable those who favour a more practical approach to increase the scientific validity of their environmental enrichment work. Ultimately, I hope this book will result in the much wider application of environmental enrichment that improves animal welfare.

Rob Young
Belo Horizonte, Brazil
February 2003

Field, D. A. (1998) ABWAK *Guidelines for Environmental Enrichment*. Top Copy, Bristol.
Shepherdson, D.J., Mellen, J.D. & Hutchins, M. (1998) *Second Nature*. p. 350. Smithsonian
    Institution Press, Washington.

Acknowledgements

In writing any book the author draws on the knowledge of his colleagues and the support of friends and family. The biggest debt of knowledge I owe is to the animal care-givers I have had the great fortune to learn from and work alongside. Two above all others whom I wish to thank are Graham Law (former keeper at Glasgow Zoo, UK) and Graham Catlow (Edinburgh Zoo, UK). It was Graham Law who showed me that the application of environmental enrichment can be undertaken using a scientific approach. I should also mention that he is one of the most inspired thinkers about environmental enrichment and consequently an excellent source of stimulating conversation, especially down the pub. It was Graham Catlow who taught me the importance of understanding the animal care-giver, and that without this understanding I would achieve nothing. His clarity of thought in terms of practical environmental enrichment for primates is, in my experience, unmatched.

I have had the good fortune to work with Valerie Hare, from The Shape of Enrichment, who has boundless energy for motivating people about the subject of environmental enrichment. I wish I could tap into her energy source.

Academically, I have had many fruitful and enjoyable discussions about environmental enrichment with Jim Anderson, Hannah Buchanan-Smith, David Field, Trevor Poole, David Shepherdson, Miranda Stevenson and Natalie Waran. Alistair Lawrence as my PhD supervisor set me on this path of interest in animal welfare – an interest that also benefited enormously from the courses I received in animal behaviour from Chris Barnard and Pete MacGregor. I owe a huge debt to the many students I have supervised over the years on environmental enrichment projects, and it is this experience that has been used to construct the content of many chapters.

This book was started while I was working at De Montfort University, Lincoln, UK (my old department is now in the University of Lincoln). At DMU, I thank Daniel Mills and Jonathan Cooper for the many conversations we had about animal welfare. I also thank all of my colleagues for their support: Gary, Jill, Joy, Sarah, Rachel, Stephen and Frank. The book was finished whilst working for my present employer PUC-Minas, to whom I am grateful for support and giving me the time to write the book. I would like to thank my colleagues for their support: Adriano, German, Hugo, Nilo, Sonia, Enemir, Thaísa, Maria Tereza and Gilmar.

I owe a debt to UFAW for suggesting me as an author, to Guy Salkeld and Antonia Seymour for being my editors at Blackwell Publishing, and to James Kirkwood, Robert Hubrecht and Elizabeth Roberts at UFAW for understanding the scientific mind!

Lastly, I would like to thank my long-suffering wife, Teresa for all her support without which nothing would have been possible.

Environmental Enrichment: an Historical Perspective

1

In 1985, the Congress of the USA passed amendments to the *Animal Welfare Act* that directed the Animal Plant and Health Inspection Service (APHIS) to promulgate regulations that provide for the psychological well-being of non-human primates (Bloomsmith *et al.*, 1991). In February 1991, the US Drug Administration/APHIS issued a final ruling that states: 'Dealers, exhibitors, and research facilities must develop, document and follow an appropriate plan for environment enhancement adequate to promote the psychological well-being of non-human primates'.

In the UK, while environmental enrichment is not a legal requirement in animal keeping institutions (i.e., farms, laboratories and zoos), it certainly helps to justify laboratory animal experiments (see Chapter 7) and in the UK, zoo visitors expect to see it being implemented (Reade & Waran, 1996). Personally, I have run workshops and courses on this subject from countries as diverse as Brazil and Russia. Television programmes about animals in the UK often feature stories about how to enrich the lives of pet species (see Chapters 7 and 13). How did we arrive at this heightened level of interest in environmental enrichment? A historical perspective is very useful on any subject matter, since knowing where we have come from often determines where we should go. However, before starting we need to define what we mean by environmental enrichment.

1.1 Definitions

'Environmental enrichment is a concept which describes how the environments of captive animals can be changed for the benefit of the inhabitants. Behavioural opportunities that may arise or increase as a result of environmental enrichment can be appropriately described as behavioural enrichment' (Shepherdson, 1994).

Alternatively, environmental enrichment is 'a process for improving or enhancing zoo animal environments and care within the context of their inhabitants' behavioral biology and natural history. It is a dynamic process in which changes to structures and husbandry practices are made with the goal of increasing behavioral choices to animals and drawing out their species appropriate behaviors and abilities, thus enhancing animal welfare'. (BHAG, 1999, provided by Valerie Hare).

1.1.1 Goals

In terms of practically implementing environmental enrichment it is easier to think of its goals rather than the various definitions that exist (see above). The goals are to:

(1)   increase behavioural diversity;
(2)   reduce the frequencies of abnormal behaviour;
(3)   increase the range or number of normal (i.e. wild) behaviour patterns;
(4)   increase positive utilisation of the environment;
(5)   increase the ability to cope with challenges in a more normal way.

(Modified after Shepherdson, 1989; Chamove & Moodie, 1990)

1.1.2 Types of enrichment

Environmental enrichment is a term that applies to heterogeneous methods of improving animal welfare that includes everything from social companionship to toys. Bloomsmith *et al.* (1991) identified five major types of enrichment, each of which can be subdivided:

(1)   Social
    (1.1)   Contact
        (1.1.1)   Conspecific (pair, group, temporary, permanent)
        (1.1.2)   Contraspecific (human, non-human)
    (1.2)   Non-contact
        (1.2.1)   (visual, auditory, co-operative device)
        (1.2.2)   (human, non-human)
(2)   Occupational
    (2.1)   Psychological (puzzles, control of environment)
    (2.2)   Exercise (mechanical devices, run)
(3)   Physical
    (3.1)   Enclosure
        (3.1.1)   Size (alteration)
        (3.1.2)   Complexity (panels for apparatus)
    (3.2)   Accessories
        (3.2.1)   Internal
            (3.2.1.1)   Permanent (furniture, bars)

(3.2.1.2)   Temporary (toys, ropes, substrates)
(3.2.2)   External (hanging objects, puzzles)
(4)   Sensory
    (4.1)   Visual (tapes, television, images, windows)
    (4.2)   Auditory (music, vocalisations)
    (4.3)   Other stimuli (olfactory, tactile, taste)
(5)   Nutritional
    (5.1)   Delivery (frequency, schedule, presentation, processing)
    (5.2)   Type (novel, variety, browse, treats)

In Chapters 8–11 I discuss all the different types of enrichment and strategies for implementing them for any species of animal held in captivity. The origins of animal keeping, animal welfare and environmental enrichment are pertinent to the types of enrichment we might use and, therefore, these subjects are discussed in the remainder of this chapter.

1.2 A Short History of Animal Keeping

The origins of zoos have been extremely well documented by Bostock (1993) in his book *Animal Rights and Zoos*. To summarise briefly, the first major collections of exotic animals were housed by the ancient Egyptians (around 3000 BC). These collections were maintained for two broad reasons: (1) many of the species kept had religious significance; (2) the possession of exotic animals was regarded as a status symbol. The use of animals as status symbols by rich and royal families across Europe and the Middle East continued until around 1800. In London, the Tower of London housed the royal family's collection of exotic animals, which had included lions and polar bears (which were often presented as gifts). Then, in the early 1800s, scientists such as Darwin started to take a serious scientific interest in the Animal Kingdom, especially in classifying animals into related groups (i.e., systematics). To facilitate their work these scientists needed large collections of different species and ones that could be easily observed (this meant small barren enclosures). It was at this time in London that the royal animal collection was moved from The Tower to Regent's Park. Sir Stamford Raffles founded London Zoo in Regent's Park in 1826. For the first twenty years of its life the zoo was only open to *bona fide* scientists before finally allowing entrance to the fee paying public. Soon after the public was given access to London Zoo, letters of complaint and criticisms of the high death rates of the animals started to appear in *The Times* newspaper. The animals were largely dying from physical health problems, such as disease. The zoo responded to the problems by increasing levels of hygiene and ensuring that all newly built enclosures could be easily cleaned (this meant hard surfaced, small barren enclosures – now referred to as hard architecture) – conditions that still exist in many zoos today despite advances in veterinary medicine and despite the work of Hagenbeck on the design of naturalistic enclosures (see below).

Unfortunately for zoo animals, zoo architecture often followed trends in human architecture. In the UK in the 1960s functionalism and constructions of reinforced concrete were in fashion for human architecture. Thus, architects such as Berthold Lubetkin were designing both high-rise flats for humans and zoo-animal enclosures (much of his work can still be seen in Dudley Zoo, UK). It was not until the 1960s with the growing interest in animal welfare (spurred on by Ruth Harrison's (1964) book *Animal Machines*, see below) and the recognition of the need for conserving species from extinction by captive breeding, that many zoos developed more animal-welfare-friendly enclosures. This is despite the fact that some zoos had for many years recognised the potential for animal suffering. The archives of Edinburgh Zoo contained copies of all the annual reports produced from 1909 (before the zoo opened) to the present day. These reports make interesting reading; I have picked out below some relevant extracts to demonstrate the evolution of zoos:

1911   A paper was presented to the zoological society which suggested that if the zoo acquired polar bears it would have to provide toys and other objects as outlets for this species' well-known playful and exploratory behaviour.

1930s   The zoological society discussed the building of a tiger enclosure with an undulating front to prevent the tigers from performing their well-known parading up and down behaviour.

1950s   The zoo received criticisms in newspapers for overcrowding in the bear enclosures.

1960s   The language in the annual reports became more scientific and the animals were no longer referred to as 'the inmates'. At the same time, animals were no longer referred to by their given names.

1973   The first environmental enrichment study was conducted in the zoo by a student (Charles Watson) from the University of Edinburgh.

1981   The chimpanzees were group-housed in a large enclosure with an artificial termite mound.

1990s   Many studies on behaviour and environmental enrichment were reported as being conducted within the zoo.

It is sobering to reflect on some of the significance of these extracts, particularly that for 1911 and the fact that most zoos did little about polar bear enrichment until the 1980s (Ames, 1993). The 1930s report is clearly an unconscious reference to stereotypic route pacing, which clearly was unpopular with the visitors or why else would the zoo seek to eliminate it. A study by Lyons *et al.* (1997) has shown that this enclosure is successful at preventing the expression of pacing behaviour but this does not mean an improvement in animal welfare (see Chapter

3). The first observations of stereotypic behaviour in zoo animals were made at this time in Germany (Meyer-Holzapfel, 1968). The reasons why ideas or information that could improve animal welfare took so long to implement are unclear. (I speculate that it probably relates to the greater public awareness of animal welfare in the 1960s, and some people have suggested that the proliferation of wildlife documentaries at this time caused a change in public attitudes. It is ironic, however, that many wildlife documentaries use zoo animals for their close-ups or when they wish for a visually spectacular behaviour pattern.)

The present trends in zoo enclosure designs in western countries tend to reflect the roles of the modern zoo, in conservation, education, research and recreation (Kreger *et al.*, 1998). For example, in the US and Europe naturalistic enclosure designs are now popular because they facilitate environmental education programmes, i.e. they place the animal in the context of its environment. Today, the conservation work of zoos is co-ordinated by national (e.g. American Zoo and Aquarium Association) and international organisations (e.g. World Zoo Organisation). The main challenge facing zoos today is to house animals in enclosures that, as Tudge (1992) put it, conserves the whole animal (i.e. behaviour as well as genes). Environmental enrichment has a significant role to play with respect to this.

Humans (*Homo sapiens*) and human ancestors (e.g. *H. habilis*, *H. erectus* and Neanderthals) have been exploiting animals for food for at least two million years. Animals were principally exploited by hunting until relatively recent times (16 000 years ago) when some modern humans desisted from their nomadic hunter-gatherer lifestyle and commenced farming in one location (Passariello, 1999). The next significant advances were made when the first animals were domesticated, since domesticated animals are much easier to manage. Domestication is basically a process whereby a species becomes adapted to living with and being managed by humans. This undoubtedly involved the selection of various behavioural, physiological and morphological traits. A key trait would be reduced fear of humans. Such traits that arose during early domestications are likely to be the by-product of the process (i.e. those sheep with less fear of humans produced the most offspring) rather than a deliberate selection policy by ancient farmers. The domestic sheep was the first food animal to be domesticated (from the Asiatic mouflon) around 9000 years ago in the Middle East. Once humans had a species 'tamed' in captivity they could then start deliberate selection for desirable characteristics, such a fast growth rate and large body size. There is evidence that sheep were being selected for particular coat characteristics 8000 years ago (Pond, 1994). The world population was five million people at the time farming of animals commenced. 8000 years later it was 500 million and during the last millennium it increased to more than five billion people, having tripled between 1900 and 2000. Over this long period of time agricultural practices gradually evolved and became more refined, and species were continuously selected for traits useful to humans, e.g. increased litter size in pigs (Pond, 1994). The next major change in agricultural practices came after 1945. During the Second World War (1939–45) the UK discovered it needed to import food from the US as it was not self-sufficient in food production. After the war politicians regarded self-sufficiency in food production as essential to national security and encouraged farmers to find methods of producing more food but on the same amount of land. This gave rise to intensive systems of animal husbandry, which have been heavily criticised for their animal welfare standards (e.g. Harrison, 1964). Food from intensive farming systems was popular with the general public because it was cheap to buy. Much of the farm animal husbandry and enclosures we have today are the result of this pressure to be self-sufficient in food. Of course, public concern has created some changes, for example, the UK ban on keeping pregnant pigs in small metal crates (tethered to the crate by a short chain) and the ban on battery-cage egg production in Switzerland. However, alternative production methods produce smaller profits (Bennett, 1997) and often a premium priced product. In the UK, the Royal Society for the Protection of Animals (RSPCA) endorses high-welfare farms with the 'Freedom Food' label allowing farmers to sell their product at a premium (Kells et al., 2001).

The first animal to be domesticated was the domestic dog, from the Asiatic wolf, around 12 000 years ago in the Middle East. The process of domestication probably started with some wolves approaching close to human settlements and being fed. Humans quickly realised that wolves could prove to be useful 'look-outs' and had the potential to help with hunting animals. Over a period of time the wild wolves became tamed and the process of domestication began. There is archaeological evidence that different breeds of dogs existed 10 000 years ago. Pet breeds of dogs almost certainly were bred from dogs kept as working animals, i.e. dogs were domesticated to work for humans and then became pets – they were not domesticated to be pets (Passariello, 1999). The ancient Egyptian pharaohs kept several breeds of dogs as long ago as 1900 BC. The Chinese emperors had the pekinese breed created for them at least one thousand years ago. There now exist more than 400 breeds of dog. Over the course of the human–dog history, the environment of the dog in western countries has become much more restrictive, i.e. most dogs are restricted to their owners' house except during exercise. However, it would be wrong to think of pet-keeping as a western-society tradition: explorers discovering and charting North and South America in the 1600s and 1700s found pet-keeping to be common among indigenous peoples. The number of exotic species being kept as pets in Western societies has been rising steadily since the 1960s. Many of these species, such as reptiles, have highly specific housing and husbandry requirements to experience a good level of animal welfare. Pets in general are the forgotten animals of public concern in animal welfare (see Chapter 7) and may experience a low level of well-being, especially psychological.

Science only started to become a major force in changing human lifestyles during the period of the Industrial Revolution (1820s onwards). It was only really with the drive to develop modern medicines that animal laboratory-houses were first established – the earliest ones were in universities that taught medicine or veterinary science. These animals were largely used in anatomical investigations. The publication of *The Origin of Species* by Charles Darwin in 1858 drew the scientific communities' attention to the fact that animals could make good models for understanding human biology. Only during the 20th century was the possibility of using drugs to cure many diseases fully realised. To do their medical research, to develop new drugs, scientists needed animals – often lots of them. The use of animals in experimentation had grown to such an extent by the 1920s that it was heavily criticised by Albert Schweitzer (1875–1965 – see below). In 1947, the Universities Federation for Animal Welfare published the first book on the management and care of laboratory animals. Today millions of animals are used each year for research in laboratory animal-houses, between three and four million in the UK alone. Laboratory animal-houses have improved greatly since the growing public awareness of animal welfare in the 1960s. However, the rate of improvement is not uniform across the globe as it tends to be society driven in those countries whose people express the most concern about animal welfare, e.g. western Europe. In the UK, the level of action against animal laboratories by animal-rights groups has forced most laboratories to be designed like fortresses, thereby denying animals the best housing conditions. For example, laboratory primates in the USA are regularly housed with extensive outdoor enclosures (Eichberg *et al.*, 1991; Kessel & Brent, 2001). This is something that cannot be done in the UK because of animal-rights activists whose actions have included taking animals from laboratories, and even releasing mink (highly destructive predators) from farms into the British countryside.

The welfare problems of captive animals are often thought to be the product of modern systems of animal housing. We never imagine that beneath the Coliseum in Rome lions paced up and down in their tiny cells, or that sheep housed in a rock-walled pen chewed each others wool, or even that the Chinese emperor's pet pekinese howled when left alone. However, animal welfare scientists know that if we recreated historical housing conditions for farm, zoo or pet animals, these animals would suffer welfare problems. Unfortunately, we have no direct evidence of the level of animal-welfare experienced by animals more than a few hundred years ago. The best indirect evidence we have are teeth wear patterns from the skulls of several-thousand-year old horses – these wear patterns are identical to those produced by modern horses when crib-biting. However, it is difficult to prove categorically that these patterns were produced by crib-biting.

1.3 Two Approaches to Environmental Enrichment

The study and implementation of environmental enrichment has been dominated by two approaches since its inception: the naturalistic approach, that relies upon creating the wild environment in captivity to provide stimulation for captive animals (Forthman-Quick, 1984; Hutchins *et al.*, 1984; O'Neill *et al.*, 1991; Ogden *et al.*, 1993; Wormell & Brayshaw, 2000), and behavioural engineering, which relies upon providing devices and machines that animals operate to receive some form of reward, usually food. Scientists who favour the different approaches have often been critical of each other (Forthman-Quick, 1984). Those who favour the naturalistic approach have suggested that the behavioural engineers only succeed in promoting the performance of abnormal behaviours. Those who favour the behavioural engineering approach have countered that the provision of natural stimuli does nothing to establish the all important connection between behaviour and its natural end point, i.e. consummatory behaviour such as feeding. Forthman-Quick (1984) has pointed out that these two approaches to environmental enrichment are not dichotomies or even opposite ends of a spectrum, merely different but compatible approaches to environmental enrichment. In truth, these approaches tend to reflect the academic backgrounds of their main proponents. The important thing is not to focus on whether one approach is better than the other but to investigate what each approach can contribute to the enrichment of the lives of captive animals.

1.3.1 Naturalistic approach

The origin of the naturalistic approach is found in the work of Carl Hagenbeck and his development of Hamburg Zoo in 1907. Hagenbeck was a great admirer of landscape paintings and wished to create large moated animal enclosures that reminded him of his favourite paintings (Tudge, 1992). Thus, the love of art created a new style of zoo animal enclosure, one that eventually lead to the naturalistic approach to environmental enrichment.

The naturalistic approach seeks to recreate a visually accurate abstract of the species' natural environment in captivity (Figure 1.1). Much animal behaviour results from the presentation of external stimuli. A wild bird sees a predator and then responds by hiding in a bush or a male fish sees a female during the breeding season and then proceeds to court her, for example. The naturalistic approach principally relies on stimulating this type of behaviour. However, it has been argued, and demonstrated experimentally, that for many of these types of behaviours out-of-sight is out-of-mind (Duncan & Petherick, 1991). Thus, how much does it matter if such behaviours are not expressed? The answer to this depends on how much internal motivation has to perform such behaviour patterns. In the case of anti-predatory behaviour it is unlikely that the animal has any internal motivation to express the behaviour, unless a predator is present. However, the performance of courtship behaviour may also depend on internal motivation, i.e. the hormonal activation of this behaviour in response to increasing day length, for example.

A considerable number of behaviour patterns result from internal stimuli. A hungry pig is motivated to express foraging behaviour but a satiated pig presented with food will not forage or feed, for example. Thus, without the presence of any

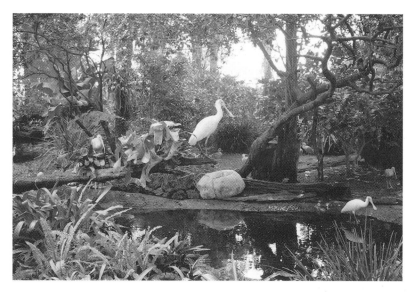

Figure 1.1 Birds in a naturalistic enclosure (© Robert J. Young).

external stimulus, animals are still motivated to express certain types of behaviour patterns, e.g. principally those behaviour patterns that restore physiological homeostasis, drinking, eating, etc. The motivation to express such behaviour patterns is only abated when the animal can express appetitive behaviour that leads to appropriate consummatory behaviour (see below).

Naturalistic environments are most important in zoos that are focussing on environmental education. The value of a naturalistic environment is that in the zoo-visitor's mind it links the animal with its natural environment (Kreger *et al.*, 1998). It is only by conserving environments that we can hope to conserve the animal species that live within them – this is the critical conservation message that zoos are trying to make.

1.3.2 Behavioural engineering

The first person to suggest the use of the behavioural engineering approach to environmental enrichment was the great primatologist Robert Yerkes. In 1925 he suggested that devices could be installed into primate enclosures that would encourage play and work. This suggestion was later repeated by Hediger in 1950 (Shepherdson *et al.*, 1998) but it was not until the 1970s that this approach was championed by Markowitz (1982). This behavioural engineering approach seeks to restore the natural contingency between the emission of appetitive behaviour (e.g. foraging) and the performance of consummatory behaviour (e.g. feeding). In 1988, Hughes and Duncan pointed to the fact that captive animals often have a need (they termed it a 'behavioural need') to express appetitive patterns of behav-

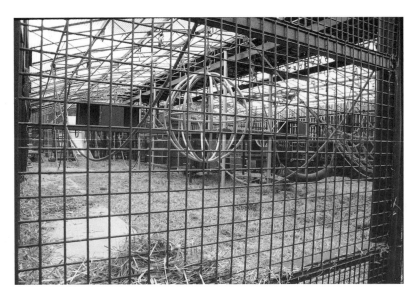

Figure 1.2 A highly artificial looking gorilla enclosure but one that is functional for the animals (© Robert J. Young).

iour. Furthermore, they suggest from their review of literature that if such a behavioural need is thwarted the welfare of the animal will suffer.

Often, environmental enrichment devices appear to be highly artificial; however, the appearance (i.e. physical form) of the behaviour expressed may be the same as if the behaviour were being naturally stimulated in the wild (Figure 1.2). Williams *et al.* (1996) used a series of wires and pulleys to make a dead rabbit move through a cheetah enclosure at high speed. The device itself looked obviously man-made but the behaviour it stimulated was completely natural looking. The problem is getting the observer to divorce the image of the enrichment device from the image of the behaviour. This is important in zoos where the use of artificial devices can dilute the educational opportunities of an enclosure (Kreger *et al.*, 1998). The physical appearance of environmental enrichment devices for laboratory, farm or pet animals is not important (except in the case of pets where it must look attractive to the buyer). Veasey *et al.* (1996b) explain that humans use running machines for exercise, these machines allow the full and natural appearance of this behaviour. In the case of animals, Young *et al.* (1994) devised a foraging device for farm-housed pigs – the device was a large white ball that dispensed food in response to natural foraging behaviour being directed at it, i.e. rooting. Of course, some environmental enrichment devices are completely artificial and have no relation to the species natural behaviour. For example, a number of primate species have been taught to play and control computer games using a joystick (Platt & Novak, 1997; Washburn *et al.*, 1994). Despite this type of environmental enrichment being completely artificial, if it improves animal welfare then that is what is important.

In highly space-restricted environments, we may be forced to use artificial devices to provide environmental enrichment, i.e. the exercise machine approach – if we put a treadmill in a tiny room the human occupant can run many miles every day. Similarly, it is often possible to install small machines in the restricted environments that exist within some laboratory animal-houses, but the use of the naturalistic approach may not be possible in such environments due to lack of space or other considerations, e.g. potential introduction of pathogens.

1.4 Animal Welfare and Environmental Enrichment

A number of different ways of defining animal welfare have been attempted. In general these definitions are separated by the emphasis that they put on different characteristics (Duncan & Fraser, 1997):

- biological functioning – the ability of the animal to function biologically within its evolutionarily selected limits;
- coping – the ability of the animal to maintain homeostasis (usually physiological) in response to environmental challenge;
- how the animal 'feels' about itself and its environment, i.e. a mentalistic approach.

From the scientific literature available on animal welfare it is possible to support any of these definitions or any combinations of these definitions. Perhaps, like environmental enrichment, we should focus on the goals of animal welfare rather than its definition since goals are more open to empirical investigation than definitions.

The basic goals of animal welfare are:

- to maintain the animal in good physical health;
- to maintain the animal in good psychological health.

As noted by Petherick and Duncan (1991), physical health and psychological health strongly interact with one another since, if an animal becomes aware of a physical health problem, this might lead to a psychological disturbance. Petherick and Duncan (1991) state that humans who discover they have a serious disease will become very worried about it, for example. Most people accept that veterinarians can measure the degree to which the physical health of an animal is being compromised. However, many of the same people would not accept that psychological health can be measured so easily and they would be correct. Even in humans it is difficult to assess psychological suffering, essentially because feelings are personal experiences that cannot be shared by anyone else (Dawkins, 1990). In

Chapters 3 and 4, I will discuss some of the tools developed and employed by scientists to assess psychological well-being.

Our attitudes to animal welfare are shaped by history, culture and society. Most societies' earliest writings about animal welfare occur in their religious books. The Old Testament, for example, states: 'Man has dominion over living things' (Genesis 1: vv. 26–7). Ancient eastern religions, such as Buddhism, are well known for the respect that they show towards animals, often based on the belief of reincarnation (which consequently influences their vegetarianism). The ancient Greek philosophers Aristotle and Pythagoras, writing hundreds of years before the birth of Christ, took different stances about animals. Pythagoras considered the killing of animals to be murder, whereas Aristotle thought that animals were god-given slaves to mankind. The Roman Empire is famous for killing animals in 'the games'; 5000 animals were slaughtered in the opening ceremonies for the Coliseum in Rome. However, there were philosophers in Roman society, such as Seneca, Plutarch and Porphyry, who criticised the slaughter of animals. From the times of the ancient Greek philosophers to 1900, animals have been tried for committing crimes – sometimes in a court with a judge, prosecution and defence council. Amusing as this observation now seems, it demonstrates that people often thought animals were culpable for their crimes and could weigh up right and wrong, i.e. the use of higher cognitive states.

From the 12th century onwards, a number of philosophers, such as St Thomas Aquinas (1225–74), Rene Descartes (1596–1650) and Gottfried Leibniz (1646–1716), were influential in proposing that God created man on a higher plane than animals, often invoking the belief that only man had a soul or only man had an 'advanced' soul. Rene Descartes proposed Cartesian dualism, essentially saying humans were composed of a body and a mind, whereas animals were only composed of a body, i.e. the separation of mental experiences from the physical body. The idea that animals only have a body has long been used as a justification for treating them without regard to their welfare. In the 18th century, the French philosopher La Mettrie (1709–51) was persecuted by the Roman Catholic Church for pointing out the similarities between humans and animals. The prevailing attitude of the Church at that time was best expressed later by Pope Pius XII (1876–1958) who considered that the cries of animals should not arouse unreasonable compassion. The destruction of Cartesian dualism by La Mettrie would, at that time, have been a threat to the Church's notion that humans were special, i.e. made in the image of God.

The first society-accepted proposals concerning the humane treatment of animals were made by the philosophers John Locke (1632–1704) and Immanuel Kant (1724–1804). They suggested that animals should be treated humanely not because of animal welfare concerns but because the mistreatment of animals brutalised society. It was the British utilitarian philosopher Jeremy Bentham (1748–1832) who put forward the following argument: 'The question is not, can they reason, nor can they talk, but can they suffer?'. Previous philosophers such as Descartes had made much of human cognitive abilities such as reasoning and language to demonstrate a significant difference between humans and animals. Thus, Bentham turned the arguments away from one of cognitive abilities to one of suffering, i.e. a move to an animal centred approach. In the UK this helped pave the way for the first animal welfare law in the world to be implemented by Richard Martin in 1826 (*The Ill treatment of Horses and Cattle Bill*). At this time in the UK, society's new attitudes to animals allowed Charles Darwin to publish his book on *The Origin of Species* (1858) that pointed out the common evolutionary history of humans and animals. In terms of considering animal welfare from a biological and therefore empirical perspective this was an important step. However, it was not until the 1960s that Ruth Harrison's book *Animal Machines* (1964) provoked the British government into commissioning large-scale empirical research into animal welfare. In her book, Harrison heavily criticised the treatment of farm animals housed under intensive systems of management. It is at this point that scientific studies into animal welfare really began. At the same time, developmental psychologists began to consider why, in their laboratories, primates exhibited strange, i.e. abnormal, behaviours (Brooman & Legge, 1997).

1.5 Developmental Psychology

Developmental psychologists in the 1960s (e.g. Harry Harlow) noticed that the primates that they housed in their laboratories developed a range of strange behaviours, such as 'floating arm syndrome'. (The arm of the primate appeaed to 'float' in the air without any conscious awareness of the primate. On occasion, primates were seen grabbing a floating arm and pulling it down.) They suspected that such behaviour might have arisen due to the ways in which the animals were housed, which was invariably in barren small cages. Therefore, they started systematically to investigate these strange behaviours by making modifications to the animals' environment by adding things. In the past they had principally measured the effects of removing things, such as light or social contact. These experiments can be regarded as the first systematic experiments of environmental enrichment (Chamove & Anderson, 1989).

1.6 The Animal Rights Movement

In the second year of my post-graduate research on farm-animal welfare, the university department in which I worked was fire bombed by the Animal Liberation Front. At the time I found it very difficult to understand why a university department in which mainly animal-welfare research was conducted would be a target for such an attack. I thought we were all working, albeit in different ways, on improving animal welfare. What I did not understand then, and many people still do not understand, are the differences between animal welfare and animal rights, and why these differences are important.

Perhaps it was Pythagoras the Greek philosopher, more famous for his geometry, who made the first known animal rights statement when he declared the killing of animals to be murder. Most animal rights supporters tend to think of Albert Schweitzer as their founding father. Working in the 1920s and 1930s he promoted the idea of reverence for all life forms and was anti animal-experimentation. In 1975 the philosopher Peter Singer published a book called *Animal Liberation* in which he proposed an idea known as 'new welfarism'. The central theme of Singer's book is that the objectives of the animal rights movement can be best met by phasing out those systems that use animals. Thus, rather than advocating immediate and total eradication of those systems that animal rights groups find objectionable he advocates a more gradual and practical solution. For example, the gradual modification of zoos until the way that they house animals means that they are no longer zoos; the animals living full natural free lives. The philosopher Tom Regan is perhaps the most well-known animal rights supporter; he argues that animals have intrinsic value that cannot be traded-off in a utilitarian analysis of animal welfare (Regan, 1984).

Anyone who works with animals in captivity (other than domestic pets) at some point will find themselves being asked to justify their keeping of animals. In many cases this will be to ensure that animals in captivity are treated ethically. Zoos, farms and laboratories often face public criticism and direct action from animal rights groups. In order to engage in a fruitful dialogue with such groups it is important to understand their perspective. The lack of fruitful discussion often results from people arguing from totally different ideological standpoints, and not appreciating this fact. For example, most people believe that animal welfare and animal rights are the same thing. However, when examined more closely they can be seen to differ fundamentally in the ways that they seek to achieve animal well-being. The purpose of this section is to summarise the differences. It should also be remembered that it is advisable that everyone who works with animals in captivity should understand and appreciate the animal rights groups' stance, since these groups are their strongest critics.

The basic animal rights stance is one in which the well-being of an animal cannot be traded-off for the greater good of mankind or for the species itself. Each individual animal has an intrinsic value that cannot have a price put on it. For example, the Director of People for the Ethical Treatment of Animals (PETA) is on record as saying that even if animal-testing produced a cure for AIDS, 'We'd be against it' (*Vogue*, September 1989). Clearly, proponents of the animal movement often believe that there can be no justification for the use of animals that in anyway compromises their well-being. Many often extend this argument to the keeping of any animals in captivity and do not accept that animal housing that does not in any way compromise animal well-being justifies the keeping of animals in captivity. The stance held by many in the animal rights movement is that all systems that impinge on the rights of animals must be eliminated.

It is important at this point to make it clear that this is an ideological and not a scientific argument. Therefore, it is often fruitless arguing with animal rights proponents about how good an environment is or how much environmental enrichment it contains. Their stand-point is that this is irrelevant as simply keeping animals in captivity is fundamentally wrong. For example, Animal Aid (who claim to be the biggest animal-rights group in the UK) have a web site (*http://www.animalaid.org.uk/*) on which there is a page titled: *The Animal Aid Awards for Mad Science 2000*. This page nominates twelve separate studies of which five are investigations into animal welfare. One study, for example, is an investigation into the very serious animal-welfare issue of animal pain: Gentle, M. J., Hocking, P. M., Bernard, R. & Dunn, L. N., (1999). Evaluation of intra-articular opioid analgesia for the relief of articular pain in the domestic fowl. *Pharmacology, Biochemistry and Behavior*, **63**, 339–43. This web page illustrates the stance of such groups to any animal research or keeping of animals in captivity.

Thus, organisations that keep animals in captivity would be far better arguing with animal rights proponents on a sociological level about the needs of human society, rather than about the details of animal housing. However, it would be fair to say that the majority of the public in most western countries do not hold such strong ideological viewpoints. In most countries people accept the need to keep animals in captivity for a variety of purposes including: food production; medical research; as pets; and in zoos for conservation efforts. For example, a MORI poll on 26th March 2000 titled *Animals in Science and Research* found that 69% of the UK public sampled would accept animal experimentation, provided that there was no unnecessary suffering. This is a high figure given the perceived stance of the UK public on animal experimentation.

Advocates of the use of environmental enrichment to improve animal well-being in captivity should realise, therefore, that animal rights groups believe that the environmental enrichment work is increasing the justification for keeping animals in captivity. It is for this reason that people working in animal welfare sometimes become targets for animal rights groups.

1.7 The Animal Welfare Movement

The adoption of an animal welfare stance means that we accept that society's use of animals is justified. This justification is normally based on two key principles:

(1) the cost in terms of animal welfare to a few animals is outweighed by the benefits obtained by the many, be they humans or animals of the same species;
(2) everything possible is done to ensure that no animals suffer unnecessarily.

Principle number one is basically a utilitarian argument, i.e. cost–benefit analysis. Thus, from this standpoint animals have a value that can be traded-off against human needs or against the needs of the species concerned as a whole. While most animal-welfare scientists accept principle one, their research is concerned with principle two, which is often enshrined in law, e.g. the UK *Animals Protection Act* (1911); *Animals (Scientific Procedures) Act* (1986). Thus, their work on principle two provides the justification for principle one. It is for this reason that some animal rights groups target animal-welfare researchers (see Animal Aid web site cited above) whom they see as justifying and perpetuating animal use. Thus, since environmental enrichment is a way of improving captive-animal welfare, it is a technique that helps justify the keeping of animals in captivity.

1.8 The Five Freedoms: a Central Concept in Animal Welfare

In an attempt to define when an animal is experiencing an acceptable level of animal welfare, the UK's Farm Animal Welfare Council (1992) developed the concept of the Five Freedoms, which are:

(1) freedom from hunger and thirst;
(2) freedom from discomfort;
(3) freedom from pain, injury and disease;
(4) freedom to express normal patterns of behaviour;
(5) freedom from fear and distress.

These Five Freedoms have also been adopted by people working with laboratory and zoo animals (Scott *et al.*, 2000) as a measure by which to judge animal welfare. The inhibition of Freedoms 1, 2, 3 and 5 would usually result in physical as well as psychological well-being problems; consequently, because of their association with physical health, they tend to be widely accepted as indicators of animal welfare (see Chapter 3). The freedom to express normal patterns of behaviour has proved more difficult to justify as an animal-welfare indicator since it often does not result in physically measurable improvements in animal welfare. The value of expressing wild behaviours to the psychological well-being of animals has been questioned (Veasey *et al.*, 1996b). However, it is not argued that expression of behaviour patterns is unimportant to animal well-being, only that not all behaviour patterns are necessary. Hughes and Duncan (1988) have demonstrated how the expression of certain behaviour patterns can represent a 'need' (a behavioural 'need') and much of current animal research is aimed at proving the value of expressing normal behaviour to animal welfare (see Chapter 3).

The approach of Scott *et al.* (2000) using the Five Freedoms in the assessment of zoo animal welfare can be used to generate questions for the inspection of animal welfare. They have expressed such questions in terms of provision rather than freedom as this is more practically orientated. I have listed (1.8.1–5) a modified form of their questions to illustrate how we might practically assess animal welfare using the concept of the Five Freedoms.

1.8.1 Provision of food and water (hunger and thirst)

(1) Is food appropriate for the species or individual supplied?
(2) Is natural feeding behaviour adequately catered for by established practices?
(3) Are feeding methods safe for staff and animals?
(4) Are supplies of food and water:
   • kept hygienically?
   • prepared hygienically?
   • supplied to the animal hygienically?
(5) Is feeding by visitors permitted and properly controlled?

1.8.2 Provision of suitable environment (discomfort)

(1) Are temperature, ventilation, lighting and noise levels appropriate?
(2) Do animal enclosures have sufficient shelter?
(3) Do animal enclosures provide sufficient space?
(4) Are back-up facilities for life support systems adequate?
(5) Is the cleaning of the accommodation satisfactory?
(6) Is the standard of maintenance of buildings and fences adequate?
(7) Is all drainage effective and safe?

1.8.3 Provision of animal health care (disease, injury and pain)

(1) Are observations of condition and health made and recorded?
(2) Do all animals receive prompt and appropriate attention when problems are noted?
(3) Are enclosures designed and operated in such a way that social interaction problems are avoided?

On-site facilities

(4) Are capture and restraint facilities adequate?
(5) Are on-site veterinary facilities adequate?
(6) Is darting equipment satisfactory?
(7) Are controlled drugs used and recorded satisfactorily?

Veterinary care

(8) Is a satisfactory programme of veterinary care established and maintained?
(9) Are appropriate veterinary records kept?
(10) Are medicines correctly kept?
(11) Are appropriate antidotes available?
(12) Are post-mortem arrangements satisfactory?

Quarantine

(13)   Is adequate reserve accommodation available for isolation of animals for assessment, treatment, recovery, etc?

Sanitation

(14)   Does it appear that general sanitation and pest control are effective?

(15)   Is transport and movement equipment in good order?

1.8.4 Provision of an opportunity to express most normal behaviour

(1)   Does accommodation appear adequately to meet the biological and behavioural needs of the animals?

(2)   Are active efforts made to enrich animal environments where necessary or advantageous?

(3)   Are enclosure barriers effective in containing animals?

(4)   Will the perimeter deter unauthorised entry and aid the confinement of zoo stock?

(5)   Are animals kept within the perimeter of the zoo?

(6)   Is captive breeding properly managed?

1.8.5 Provision of protection from fear & distress

(1)   Are animals handled only by, or under the supervision of appropriately qualified staff?

(2)   Is physical contact between animals and the public consistent with the animals' welfare?

(3)   Are interactions between animals such that they are not excessively stressful?

It is useful to reflect upon these questions because they illustrate the importance of good human management of animals to ensure that high levels of animal welfare are attained.

1.9 Animal Welfare Indicators

Broom (1999) has produced a list of measures of poor animal welfare:

- reduced longevity;
- reduced ability to grow or breed;
- body damage (i.e. injury);
- disease;
- immunosuppression;
- physiological attempts to cope;
- behavioural attempts to cope;

- behaviour pathology (e.g. stereotypies, apathy, self-mutilation, learned helplessness);
- self narcotisation;
- extent of behavioural aversion expressed;
- extent of the suppression of normal behaviour patterns;
- extent to which normal physiological processes and anatomical development are inhibited.

Broom (1999) has also produced a list of good welfare measures:

- variety of normal behaviours expressed;
- extent to which strongly preferred behaviours can be expressed;
- physiological indicators of pleasure;
- behavioural indicators of pleasure.

The scientific validity of these measures as welfare indicators, their practical application and other problems associated with their use are discussed in Chapter 3.

1.10 Conclusion

In this chapter I have tried to set the rest of the book in context: I have done this principally through brief histories of subjects that pertain to environmental enrichment. The reasons why history is so important as a subject are that it provides us with the opportunity to learn from the mistakes of others and that it enables us to understand why people and societies hold differing view-points on a subject. My professional experience has taught me that these two points are critical when working in an emotive subject. Furthermore, I believe that arguing about definitions when working in an applied science is 'to fiddle while Rome burns': much more can be achieved by having specific goals (see enrichment goals above).

Why Bother with Environmental Enrichment?

It might seem a strange question to pose in a book about environmental enrichment but anyone who works in institutions with animals will no doubt have heard: 'Why should I use environmental enrichment?'

2.1 Why Use Enrichment?

Let us look first at the 'why not' and the types of arguments used against the application of environmental enrichment:

- it increases the costs of maintaining animals in captivity;
- it creates additional work for animal caregivers;
- it creates a more risky environment for animals;
- it increases variability in experimental animals;
- there is no scientific proof that it improves animal welfare.

Undoubtedly, the application of environmental enrichment can increase the costs of maintaining animals in captivity. However, the cost of well thought-out enrichment programmes should be minimal. In addition to the costs of environmental enrichment we must look at how they are offset by benefits (for an example see Chamove & Anderson, 1989). In a zoo, environmental enrichment might well enhance visitor satisfaction, however, benefits such as this are difficult to measure (certainly hard to incorporate into an accountant's spreadsheet). In the laboratory, the application of environmental enrichment might increase the number of customers who wish to use your laboratory for their research, especially as many laboratories are now contract houses. On the farm, environmental enrichment might allow you to sell your product as welfare friendly and, therefore, at a premium price (Webster, 2001). In the home, environmental enrichment might enhance your relationship with your pet, again something that cannot be analysed financially. Therefore, in a cost–benefit analysis we might well find that environmental enrichment increases our 'net profit' (see Chamove & Anderson, 1989).

2.1.1 The cost of enrichment

The cost of human labour is one of the highest expenditures in most companies and, therefore, companies try to minimise labour force size (Waterhouse, 1996; Reinhardt & Roberts, 1997). Much environmental enrichment can be built into an enclosure when it is first constructed (see Chapter 10) and this will not use any staff time. Institutions have, of course, the power to chose the types of enrichment they use. Therefore, if staff time is at a premium they need to use non-labour-intensive methods or look at other solutions (see Chapter 1). One of the most popular solutions is the use of environmental enrichment volunteers (Bloomsmith et al., 1991). A number of zoos around the world, and at least a few laboratories in the US, actively use enrichment volunteers. These volunteers collect the materials from which the environmental enrichment is going to be made, and usually make the environmental enrichment. However, they must not be allowed to place it within animal enclosures, as this would contravene health and safety standards in most countries. Furthermore, it is then difficult for the animal care-givers to monitor and manage the enrichment programme (see Chapter 6) of their institution. Thus, we need to implement the adage: 'we need to work smarter not harder'.

Personally, I know of only three documented cases of environmental enrichment causing physical well-being problems (Hahn et al., 2000; Shomer et al., 2001; Bazille et al., 2001). In addition to these records, I have informally been told about a number of accidents and even deaths of animals that have resulted from environmental enrichment. The common thread linking all these accounts is that the institution concerned did not implement properly a safety evaluation programme (see Chapter 5). Of course, some accidents are unpredictable or freak occurrences but these are rare. I would strongly argue that environmental enrichment that has been properly safety evaluated increases the risk of accidents by an infinitesimally small amount. Given the benefits that animals receive from environmental enrichment I think we can dismiss this argument, as the 'net profit' for the animals is huge (see below and Chapter 3).

2.2 Justifying Enrichment

The guiding principles of laboratory animal research developed by William Russell and Rex Birch at UFAW in the 1950s are the three Rs, replacement, reduction and refinement (Russell, 1995). Refinement often is equated with environmental enrichment. Normally, in laboratory animal research, the objective is to minimise all sources of variation to achieve highly accurate and reliable results. It could be argued that environmental enrichment that empowers animals to express behaviour patterns as they wish introduces variation. Especially given that animals are not clones, therefore, we will see some individual differences, that could potentially generate some variation in certain types of data, e.g. behavioural data. This is not necessarily a bad thing, such variation can elucidate the evolution of different behavioural strategies, for example. As mentioned previously, in laboratory studies of toxicology, the possibility of variation is undesirable. However, if the enrichment means that a chemical is being tested on a non-stressed and healthy animal then the results are more reliable (see Tables 3.1–3.3). The purpose of toxicity testing is usually to establish if the chemical is toxic in healthy animals. It would be naive to deny that a badly thought out and poorly implemented environmental-enrichment programme could cause confounding variation in some experimental studies. The solution to this problem is education, not the rejection of environmental enrichment (van Zutphen & van der Valk, 2001; Smaje et al., 1998; Orlans, 1996).

Environmental enrichment is perhaps unique in animal welfare in that there has been more application than scientific evaluation of its effects on animal welfare, especially in zoos and laboratories. However, we now have a large number of empirically validated studies that demonstrate the animal welfare benefits of environmental enrichment, these are reviewed in Chapter 3 (see Tables 3.1–3.3). If one wishes to be ultra cautious, then only implement those types of enrichment that have been empirically validated. However, I believe to do so would be to deny animals access to a greater range of enrichment and it would undoubtedly de-motivate animal care-givers (see Chapter 6).

2.3 The Ethical Imperative for Environmental Enrichment

Animal welfare and ethics are inextricably linked together (Bostock, 1993; Norton et al., 1995; Fraser et al., 1997; Kreger et al., 1998; Holst, 1998). Ethics is the scientific study of morals: morals are what society considers good (and, therefore, acceptable) and bad (therefore unacceptable; see Sandøe et al., 1997). In human society we believe that medical patients should receive the best care available and to give them inferior treatment is unethical, for example. Ethically, if we know of ways to improve the psychological as well as the physical well-being of animals, I believe we are ethically bound to take them. I am not denying that ethics work within constraints. Returning to our human patient, if our patient had a rare disease that could be partially treated at the cost of a million pounds society might find this acceptable, but if the cost of the best treatment for this patient was 500 billion pounds society would probably find this unacceptable. Thus, in a practical sense, ethics really is about what society deems acceptable. Given that I have already demonstrated that the cost–benefits of environmental enrichment usually result in 'net profit', I think it is unethical not to implement environmental enrichment, but I am not saying that this is always easy. (See Chapter 7 for discussion of constraints and restriction on implementing environmental enrichment for companion, farm, laboratory and zoo animals.) Here I am using a utilitarian standpoint to justify my ethical stance. Of course, it is possible, as animal rights activists do, to use a different philosophical standpoint (Sandøe *et al.*, 1997). However, as I believe that the use of animals and the maintenance of animals in captivity is important for animals and humans, I am only concerned with a utilitarian standpoint. (See Chapter 1 for a further discussion of animal welfare versus animal rights.)

2.3.1 Public pressure for enrichment

One of the most powerful vehicles of change is public pressure (Howkins & Merricks, 2000; Pocard, 1999; Odberg, 1996; Matfield, 1995). This is especially relevant when there is a direct connection between the public and the institution that they wish changed. In terms of animal-using institutions, zoos are perhaps the only institution that the public can directly affect financially, simply by not visiting the institution. Many zoos around the world are, to a great extent, dependent on visitor fees to survive. In the UK, zoos exist almost exclusively on this income; in contrast, in Brazil many zoos are 80–100% funded by federal institutions. Thus, power of direct public pressure varies around the world, as of course do public attitudes to animal welfare (Kohn, 1994; Odberg, 1996; Knierim & Jackson, 1997; Holst, 1998; Balls, 1999). For example, within western Europe some believe that there is a geographical variation in animal welfare, with countries in the north being more concerned than those in the south.

In most countries around the world there are people who are very concerned about animal welfare, what varies is the level of public concern. I believe that it is this direct public financial connection that has been a great motivator to reform the animal-welfare standards within zoos around the world. Reade and Waran (1996) conducted a survey of UK zoo visitors' expectations. Over 90% of visitors expected animal welfare and environmental enrichment to be a priority of the zoo and expected to see evidence of its implementation. Of course, a criticism of this survey is that it only represents zoo visitors, not a sample of the general population. Many television companies now make or have made series about the life of animals within a zoo (e.g., in the UK the BBC series *Zoo Keepers*), however, there are no series about farm (the comedy film *Chicken Run* being something of an exception) or laboratory animals, only the occasional documentary.

Surveys suggest that 600 million people, or 10% of the world's population, visit zoos every year (Whitehead, 1995). In contrast, the number of people that now visit farms, especially in Western society, or laboratories is minuscule. Most of the global population is completely unaware of how laboratory animals are housed. In the developed world most people have no idea of how farm animals are housed or their food produced. Thus, there is no direct connection between the public and these institutions, instead, most people's connection is through intermediary organisations, supermarkets and pharmacists. Added to this, most developed societies use distancing devices to make the consumption of such products more palatable.

Meat is usually presented to the consumer in a manner that makes no connection with its animal of origin (e.g. the packaging does not contain a picture of the species) and in most languages we do not say 'dead pig meat' we use a neutral term, such as 'bacon' or 'pork' (Serpell, 1999). It is little wonder, given these conditions, that the public are less motivated to effect changes in the housing of farm and laboratory animals.

I am not denying that there is considerable public concern in many countries around the world about laboratory animal welfare. Those people who oppose the use of laboratory animals are, perhaps, the most vocal of all animal rights protesters (Howkins & Merricks, 2000; Bekoff, 1997; Bostock, 1993; Spira, 1991; Regan, 1984). However, the activists are a minority of the population. Government-commissioned surveys in the UK by MORI in 1998, for example, show that while the public are concerned about animal experimentation most of them perceive it to be necessary. The level of misinformation concerning the housing and use of laboratory animals is perhaps one of the greatest problems facing the public. The media tend to portray laboratories in a negative light. For example, a government research institute opened a new laboratory primate house in the UK a few years ago, the facility was state-of-the-art and included features such as group housing. The institution invited the media to the opening and the next day one national newspaper covered the opening with a photograph of a singly-housed primate in a small cage, under the photograph in tiny typeface was the comment that this was not the institution. Clearly, this newspaper wished to portray this institution in a negative light. Given this bias it is hard to see how better information about laboratory animals will become available to the public.

2.3.2 The legal imperative for enrichment

Most countries around the world have minimum legal standards for the housing of laboratory animals, a considerable number also have such regulations for farm animals, very few countries have regulations concerning zoo animals, and virtually no countries have legislation concerning the housing of companion animals (Meyer, 2000; Pocard, 1999; Knierim & Jackson, 1997; Baumgartner, 1994). (Although, most countries have anti-cruelty laws, e.g. the UK *Animals Protection Act* 1911 and subsequent amendments, this mainly protects physical well-being; i.e. the prevention of cruelty not mental suffering.) Where legislation exists, it is obviously a persuasive reason to implement environmental enrichment, provided that the law is enforceable and is enforced within the country concerned. To be enforceable a law needs to be written clearly with no ambiguous terms. In the US, the law requiring environmental enrichment for captive primates (see Chapter 1) used the term 'psychological well-being' and a number of opponents of this law have tried to argue that no scientific consensus about this term exists, therefore, the law is un-implementable. Enforcement of a law requires the government to appoint an organisation, such as the police, or to create a special organisation (inspectorate) with the powers to enforce it (Brooman & Legge, 1997).

In the UK laboratory animal houses may have a greater chance of having their experimental protocol approved if they can demonstrate the implementation of the highest animal-welfare standards, including the use of environmental enrichment. Thus, although laboratories are not directly legislated to implement enrichment, there is considerable pressure to do so. In Europe, there are moves to create European-wide legislation concerning the standards of housing and welfare for zoo animals. The UK has already produced a document that outlines proposed new animal-welfare standards for zoos (see Scott *et al.*, 2000); the welfare section of this document is based on FAWC's concept of the Five Freedoms (Hughes, 1996). The Secretary of State's Standards of Modern Zoo Practice were published in 2000 and are available, with advice from the Zoo Forum, on the DEFRA website. In terms of farm animal welfare, the UK Department of Environment, Food and Rural Affairs (DEFRA) produces a series of leaflets on the welfare of farm animal species (see Chapter 13 for details). These leaflets provide advice to farmers on how to house and care for their animals in such a manner that, if they follow the advice within, they are unlikely to break the law. They operate on the same principle as the *Highway Code*, which informs drivers how to behave when driving so that they are unlikely to break the law, but without explicitly stating each law. These information books are often referred to as deregulated legislation (Knierim & Jackson, 1997). Unfortunately, the present leaflets on animal housing do not directly mention environmental enrichment, but clearly they are a legal device the UK Government could use in the future.

Legislating to improve the welfare of pets, I feel, is the greatest animal-welfare challenge society faces and few studies have been conducted into pet welfare (Schuppli & Fraser, 2000; Anon., 1999; Bride, 1998; Podberscek, 1997; Wegner, 1993; Kamphues, 1993). Currently, many countries have excellent anti-animal cruelty laws that protect the physical well-being of animals (see above) and laws governing pets in shops (Moritz, 2000; Bollhofer, 1996; Nowak, 1993). Prosecution under these laws often requires that a veterinary surgeon states that the animal was subjected to 'unnecessary suffering' and few veterinary surgeons are prepared to make such statements in relation to psychological suffering. Until we can cross this impasse the psychological well-being of pets is likely to remain the least protected area of animal welfare. It is, of course, difficult to imagine how we could implement and enforce laws on the psychological well-being of pets. A starting point might be to give them the same animal-welfare standards as their conspecifics receive when housed in laboratories, zoo or farms, depending on which has the highest welfare standards. The paradoxical treatment of captive animals and especially pet animals never fails to amaze me.

Let us take the rabbit as an example. In the UK, there is legislation stating the minimum cage size for a rabbit housed in a laboratory (where females are often group housed in large rooms) and for one housed on a farm. However, no such legislation exists for the housing of pet rabbits. Austen (1994), conducted a survey of the sizes of rabbit cages and hutches available for sale in UK pet shops. Her results showed that pet shops were selling cages and hutches below the legal minimum sizes for laboratory- and farm-housed rabbits. Also, that rabbits in laboratories had the largest legally required cage size and that if they were housed in farm-sized cages this would have broken the law. A possibly greater paradox is that it is very rare for dogs to be solitary housed within UK laboratories and yet many pet dogs are left alone for many hours of each day (Simpson, 2000; Flannigan & Dodman, 2001). Although we may not be able to implement animal welfare standards as easily in peoples homes, we can at the very least be consistent in the treatment of a species and employ the highest legislated animal welfare standards that exist. For example, make it illegal for pet shops to sell rabbit cages or hutches that are smaller than the minimum standard required under law for laboratory rabbits.

I for one am not suggesting that legislation is the best way to promote animal welfare. Personally, I believe education is the best way to promote good standards of animal welfare. The problem with legislation is that it usually states a set of minimum standards, cage size, for example. These minimum standards rather than being an extreme part of the normal distribution of housing standards observed usually become the mean, the median and the mode. The space allowance for battery hens being a case in point; nearly all hens in the UK receive the statutory minimum standard of $450\,cm^2$ (Appleby *et al.*, 1992). In the laboratory-animal industry, the legislation concerning minimum standards has been more prone to changes and as a consequence institutions have tended to future-proof their financial investment in animal housing by constructing housing that is well beyond the minimum standards. Unfortunately, more minimum standards, such as those produced by DEFRA, in the UK, and other organisations are too simplistic and often only focus on things that will affect physical well-being, such as stocking density or space allowance. Animals do have a requirement for a minimum amount of space (see Chapter 1) but, as I have argued before about this minimum, it is quality of space that is important. In Norway, the government has implemented a law that all captive bears must receive a minimum space allowance of $30\,000\,m^2$ but if the animal's enclosure is $30\,000\,m^2$ of bare concrete, then probably it would experience the same level of animal welfare in an enclosure one tenth of the size.

The relationship between the implementation of animal-welfare standards and legislation is a complex one. In many countries legislation can be driven by the public, if the public exert sufficient pressure on politicians it is often possible to get a government to consider implementing new legislation. However, the actual enshrining of public concerns within legislation is, even in most democracies, not a straightforward process. In the UK, the vast majority of the public have wished to see the end of fox hunting with dogs for a great many years (see *http://www.huntinginquiry.gov.uk*) but over the years various legal and political devices have been used to stall the legislative process (Note: In 2002 the Scottish Parliament banned fox hunting).

2.3.3 Self-regulation and the implementation of enrichment

A route similar to legislation, is the control of animal-welfare standards by the professional body representing the member institutions. In the US, most of the major zoos are members of the American Zoo and Aquarium Association (AZA). This association has rules that its members must follow to maintain their membership. Zoos gain considerable public respect in the US from being AZA members, consequently, membership is something they are motivated to maintain. Thus, organisations such as AZA have the power to effect some control over the animal-welfare standards of their member institutions. The AZA is concurrently considering implementing rules that will commit members to implementing environmental enrichment with every species they house. This type of control over standards is sometimes referred to as self-regulation. The *Freedom Foods* brand endorsed and regulated by the RSPCA (Kells *et al.*, 2001) is another example of this type control of using non-legislative rules. Clearly, well organised professional bodies do have the power to exert control over the standards used by their members. (Obviously, they need a method of inspection and enforcement.)

2.4 Zoos: a Special Case for Enrichment

While zoos often talk about reintroduction programmes as being their ultimate goal for conservation, the most important conservation function of most zoos is the creation of safety-net populations through captive breeding (Tudge, 1992). Seidensticker and Doherty (1996) have argued that zoos must not only maintain species genetic material into future generations but also maintain individuals' behavioural competence, i.e. the maintenance of key survival skills. The ultimate test of an animal's behavioural competence is re-introduction. Evidence presented by Castro *et al.* (1998) on golden lion tamarins seems to suggest that animals reared in enriched environments had no better survival skills than those reared in conventional environments. However, the authors concede that the high number of confounding variables (e.g. rearing history of individual animals) makes drawing any reliable conclusion about the effect of enrichment on survival at reintroduction difficult: I think we will just have to wait for more data. The authors of this study found that golden lion tamarins reared in conventional zoo enclosures had the full behavioural repertoire of their wild conspecifics. However, they believe that they lack refined survival skills (i.e. the efficiency of many behaviour patterns was less than that of their wild counterparts) and that these could potentially be developed within an enriched environment, for example, a free-range environment.

Castro *et al.* (1998) were clearly referring to an often missed or ignored part of behavioural expression – the quality of the behaviour expressed. Scattering food in a large enclosure can create a foraging time budget for captive chimpanzees that is identical to their conspecifics. However, wild conspecifics do not simply walk from place to place picking up food, they often use complex food processing skills, e.g. removing the skin of fruits or cracking nuts open with stones. Byrne (2001) has conducted studies that show that even the feeding behaviour of mountain gorillas consists of a series of complex manipulations of the food and such skills take time to learn.

The work of Miller *et al.* (1998) and Castro *et al.* (1998) has clearly demonstrated that it is possible to train and improve the efficiency of animal survival skills, while they are within a captive environment. Brown and Laland (2001) have reviewed studies on the survival skills of hatchery reared fish showing that they too lack behavioural competence and that it should be possible to train animals to develop these skills. It may, however, be the case that to train animals in survival skills we need to expose them to very stressful and dangerous situations (see Castro *et al.*, 1998; Miller *et al.*, 1998). In the case of the black-footed ferret, ground predator avoidance skills were trained by having muzzled dogs chase the animals (Miller *et al.*, 1998), a situation that would be illegal in many countries. It might be only this kind of extreme experience that actually has the ability to make an animal's survival skills effective. Certainly, successful reintroduction of carnivores only occurs when they have experience of hunting and killing live prey (Young, 1997). It would be fair to say that our present understanding of the interaction between enriched environments and the development of survival skills is limited. An excellent discovery to illustrate this is the study by Masataka (1993) who found that exposure to live insects activated snake fear in squirrel monkeys, a discovery that no one would have predicted.

In many cases, environmental enrichment reduces stress, which can interfere with the reproductive process (Schuett, 1996; Kleiman, 1994; Carlstead & Shepherdson, 1994). Environmental enrichment can also create an environment in which an animal is motivated to give birth (see Chapter 3). It should be noted that in general species that are k-selected (i.e. those whose reproductive strategy is to produce a few large altricial offspring) are normally more difficult to breed in captivity than r-selected species (i.e. those who produce many small precocial offspring). Further, many species of farm animal have been under extreme selection pressure to have high fecundity, irrespective of housing conditions (Fregonesi & Leaver, 2001). However, environmental enrichment has been shown to increase profitability in egg production in battery hens by increasing food conversion efficiency (Bell & Adams, 1998). Thus, in organisations that are trying to breed animals, for whatever purpose, environmental enrichment can help them achieve their goals.

The educational value of animals within zoos is directly related to them expressing normal patterns of behaviour. Education programmes in zoos normally focus on environmental education and they need good exemplars of the species concerned. It is difficult to teach children about the adaptations of a tiger when the animal in the enclosure in front of them is pacing up and down. Kreger *et al.* (1998) have reviewed the literature concerning the aesthetics of animal presentation and education. The aesthetics of presentation not only concerns how the animals' enclosures appear visually but also the visual appearance of animals' behaviour. The message conveyed by a stereotyping animal against the backdrop of a naturalistic enclosure is a confused one. Perhaps more confusing is the use of man-made objects (e.g. the ubiquitous traffic cone) in a naturalistic enclosure. Environmental enrichment can, therefore, be used to promote the expression of natural behaviour patterns in a natural time budget. Promoting the hunting behaviour of carnivores through enrichment (e.g. (Markowitz, 1982; Markowitz *et al.*, 1995; Williams *et al.*, 1996) is not only good for animal welfare but provides an opportunity for zoo visitors to learn more about such a species' abilities. Demonstrating the spectacular abilities of animals can only help to increase public admiration of them. Thus, environmental enrichment has much to contribute to the education of the zoo-going public.

2.5 Care-givers and Enrichment

In Chapter 9 I discuss at some length the benefit of the human–animal bond to solitary housed animals. Over the years, a number of articles have appeared in the magazine *The Shape of Enrichment* as to whose life is enriched by environmental enrichment. The answer is simple, the animal and its care-givers. Here I will focus on the enrichment of the care-givers' life. In nearly all types of organisation the animal care-givers' work has principally consisted of feeding the animals and cleaning out their enclosures. This type of work is, to say the least, somewhat repetitive and boring for the care-giver. Introducing environmental enrichment for the animals under their care introduces variation to the animal care-givers' work. It should provide them with the opportunity to think about how to enrich the lives of the animals they look after, and to perform the new tasks associated with enrichment. Potentially, environmental enrichment should add the following tasks to the care-givers' work: researching the species, finding the materials for the enrichment, constructing the enrichment, monitoring the enrichment and recording the enrichment.

All these tasks help to empower the care-giver (see Chapter 6). It is little wonder that the vast majority of animal care-givers believe that environmental enrichment actually enriches their life. Hemsworth and Gonyou (1997) have discussed the value of having animal care-givers (in his studies, stockhands) that are happy in their job. They found that happy care-givers are more likely to interact in a positive way with their animals and by having a happy frame of mind they are much more predictable; lack of predictability in animal care-givers' behaviour is known to be a major source of stress for animals. One must never forget that good animal husbandry and animal welfare are totally dependent on good management of animal care-givers.

2.6 Conclusion

The benefits that can be derived from environmental enrichment depend on why the animal is being kept in captivity in the first place. However, all animals, irrespective of their category, will receive welfare and reproductive benefits. Society generally accepts the use of animals by humans within the utilitarian framework of cost–benefit analysis of animal welfare (see Chapter 1). Thus, environmental enrichment helps to reduce the cost in terms of animal welfare, thereby increasing the cost–benefit ratio such that the benefits outweigh the costs. Thus, environmental enrichment is an important factor allowing humans ethically to continue using animals for their benefit. In many cases of animal use, environmental enrichment may increase financial profitability (Bell & Adams, 1998) or at the very least enhance the ability of the organisation to achieve its goals (Kreger et al., 1998).

Does Environmental Enrichment Work?

It is often assumed, quite wrongly, that something that has good intentions for animal welfare must result in a positive improvement. However, in science we cannot rely on good intentions, we need scientific proof. It is possible, for example, that certain forms of environmental enrichment may actually decrease the welfare of animals. Therefore, it is useful to review the empirical evidence that environmental enrichment improves animal welfare. I should also state at the outset that many of the measures of animal welfare are still being developed and what they actually measure is sometimes disputed in the scientific literature (e.g. see Appleby & Hughes, 1997). Therefore, I will present scientific evidence with which the majority of animal-welfare researchers would agree, but not all. It is useful to reflect that in science we rely on statistical proof – nothing is 100% certain. For the sake of brevity, I have summarised the arguments concerning the use of different evidence as animal welfare indicators but I strongly recommend that the interested reader consults the research papers I have cited. (For an introduction to animal welfare I recommend Appleby & Hughes, 1997.)

3.1 The Evidence

There are three main lines of evidence used to test whether environmental enrichment actually improves animal welfare, these are: behavioural, physiological and neurological. An important point to note is that there are virtually no data from studies of companion animals. The data available on the physiological and neurological studies are almost exclusively from studies of farm and laboratory animals. The zoo literature contains large numbers of studies using behavioural evidence because this information is easy to obtain and does not require central government licensing in most countries. However, many of the studies conducted on zoo animals have used sample sizes too small for statistical analysis (often N = 1), which authors have overcome by pseudo-replication (e.g. Williams *et al.*, 1996; see section 12.2.3 for further discussion) and pooling data from animals kept in groups (Ings *et al.*, 1997; see also Chapter 12). The implications of this are that it is difficult to generalise the effects reported in such studies to other animals.

3.1.1 The behavioural evidence

The behavioural evidence that environmental enrichment improves animal welfare is detailed in Table 3.1. In this table I have only included experimental studies that have been published in peer-reviewed journals. In many cases the enrichment study improved several aspects of animal welfare, e.g. a reduction in feather pecking and an increase in foraging behaviour. In these cases I chose what I considered to be the most important measure of welfare improvement; in the aforementioned case this would be the reduction in feather pecking (reduction of injurious behaviour). I have explicitly excluded studies that only consider the usage of an enrichment device or technique.

The main measures of animal welfare improved by environmental enrichment, from Table 3.1, are: reduction in the performance of abnormal behaviour (Figure 3.1), the expression of 'desirable' behaviour patterns, and reductions in the expression of injurious or aggressive behaviour. However, from Table 3.1 we can see that environmental enrichment can improve the welfare (behaviour) of animal species

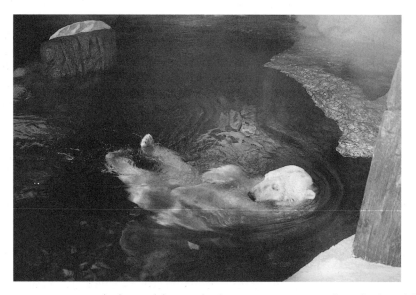

Figure 3.1 A captive polar bear exhibiting a back-swimming stereotypy; this polar bear follows the exact swimming route for hours (© Robert J. Young).

in a broad variety of ways. I should point out that the data in Table 3.1 are not definitive, nor can they be because of the large number of unpublished studies that exist; this is especially a problem with experiments that produced either neutral or negative results.

There are a few published studies that demonstrate either a negative or a neutral effect of environmental enrichment on behaviour measures of animal welfare. Principally, such studies have reported an increase in aggression due to environmental enrichment (e.g. McGregor & Ayling, 1990). The underlying cause of the aggression in such studies is often due to environmental enrichment facilitating the expression of territorial behaviour, e.g. in fish (Nijman & Heuts, 2000) or mice (Nevison et al., 1999). The enrichment either acts as territorial markers or as a resource of high value that is defendable. In the studies where the enrichment became a resource of high value, the solution is obvious – provide sufficient enrichment for all individuals to have simultaneous access. A few documented studies have recorded an accident involving an enrichment device (see Chapter 5). The neutral results obtained usually are in studies of farm animals (Sherwin, 1993) or in caged animals (Line et al., 1991). It is difficult to generalise why some farm animal experiments into environmental enrichment produced neutral results. One negative result for human care-givers is that environmental enrichment can reduce the animals' fear of humans to such a degree that they become difficult to handle (Day et al., 2002).

We should of course question how reliable and accurate the behavioural measures reported in Table 3.1 are in relation to animal welfare. Hughes and Duncan (1988) described the fulfilling of motivational or 'behavioural needs' to be essential to good animal welfare. In their literature review, they concluded that the thwarting of a behavioural need (e.g. a hungry pig expressing foraging behaviour) often caused measurable animal-welfare problems, such as the performance of abnormal behaviour. The performance of abnormal behaviour by captive animals is widely used as an animal-welfare indicator (for a discussion, see Mason, 1991) and there is a considerable amount of supporting behavioural and physiological evidence to support its use as an animal-welfare indicator (Lawrence & Rushen, 1993). However, it would be wrong to say that the performance of abnormal behaviour is a definitive animal-welfare indicator. Research is still continuing into its exact value as an animal-welfare indicator. If we know the causation of the abnormal behaviour then I believe we can use this animal-welfare indicator with some confidence. For example, if the abnormal behaviour is a laying hen pacing in a battery cage for the hour before it is due to lay its eggs, we know that the abnormal behaviour is caused by frustration.

The reduction of injurious behaviour, such a feather pecking in birds, tail biting in pigs or piglet crushing by sows, obviously results in an increase in the animals' physical well-being. I believe, therefore, such changes associated with environmental enrichment undeniably represent an improvement in animal welfare. The reduction in fear levels and reactivity to stressors, are considered to be one of the

Table 3.1 Behavioural evidence that environmental enrichment improves animal welfare.

Measure of improvement	Species	References
Meets behavioural needs of the animal, i.e. fulfils motivational requirements (for discussion see Hughes & Duncan, 1988).	Giant pandas, sows (female pigs).	Swaisgood et al., 2001; Damm et al., 2000; Thodberg et al., 1999.
Reduction of abnormal behaviour such as stereotypies.	Seals, horses, rabbits, wood rats, mice, baboons, chimpanzees, leopards, rhesus macaques, bears.	Grindrod & Cleaver, 2001; Henderson & Waran, 2001; Hansen & Berthelsen, 2000; Lidfors, 1997; Callard et al., 2000; Wurbel et al., 1998; Brent & Belik, 1997; Baker, 1997; Markowitz et al., 1995; O Neill et al., 1991; Carlstead et al., 1991.
Reduction of injurious behaviour, e.g. feather pecking in birds or sows crushing piglets.	Turkeys, pigs, hens, non-human primates, conures (parrot species).	Martrenchar et al., 2001; Sherwin et al., 1999b; de Jong et al., 2000b; Bubier, 1996; Norgaardnielsen et al., 1993; Holmes et al., 1995; van Hoek & King, 1997.
Reduction of fear and reactivity to stressors, e.g. being handled.	Chicks (hens), rats, broilers, hens, pigs, mice.	Clarke & Jones, 2000; Zimmermann et al., 2001; Nicol, 1992; Reed et al., 1993; Hubrecht, 1993; Day et al., 2002; Lemercier, 2000; Van de Weerd et al., 1994.
Promotion of natural time-budgets (for discussion see Veasey et al., 1996b).	Fruit bats, horses, pigs.	O'Connor, 2000; Winskill et al., 1996; Beattie et al., 1996; Young et al., 1994.

Reduction in aggressive behaviour.	Oryx (desert antelope), pigs, lemurs, stump-tailed macaques, chimpanzees.	Patton et al., 2001; Beattie et al., 2000a; Beattie et al., 2000b; O'Connell & Beattie, 1999; Zimmermann & Feistner, 1996; Estep & Baker, 1991; Brent & Eichberg, 1991.
Protection against cognitive defects caused by stressors (e.g. handling), diet (e.g. high fat) or age.	Rats.	Pham et al., 1999b; Winocur & Greenwood, 1999; Soffie et al., 1999; Escorihuela et al., 1994.
Increases behavioural diversity.	Capuchins, leopard cats.	Ludes-Fraulob & Anderson, 1999; Shepherdson et al., 1993.
Increases space utilisation.	Rhesus macaques, cheetahs.	Lutz & Novak, 1995; Williams et al., 1996.
Promotion of behaviour patterns (i.e. foraging, exploration, activity and play) that are perceived as 'desirable' by the scientific community.	Fruit bats, broilers, rhesus macaques, bush dogs, cats, Jamaican boas, rats, pigs, bears, dogs.	Masefield, 1999; Kells et al., 2001; Platt & Novak, 1997; Ings et al., 1997; de Monte & LePape, 1997; Cardiff, 1996; Van Waas & Soffie, 1996; Arey & Maw, 1995; Fischbacher & Schmid, 1999; Hubrecht, 1993.
Control over the environment.	Macaque species.	Vick et al., 2000.
Increased learning ability.	Rats.	Tees, 1999a; Gomez-Pinilla et al., 1998; Passig et al., 1996.

basic freedoms that an animal in captivity should possess (i.e. the Five Freedoms; Webster, 2001; Hughes, 1996). Many animals experience frightening events, such as being handled, that have no negative impact on them except for the process itself. Thus, the elimination or reduction of unnecessary fear represents an important improvement in animal welfare.

The promotion of a natural time-budget has proven popular in the past as an animal-welfare indicator but there are a number of theoretical and practical objections to its use. For example, the time-budget expressed by an animal is usually a reflection of resource (e.g. food, water, shelter, companions, etc.) density and distribution. Furthermore, the duration or frequency of a behaviour tells us nothing about the importance of that behaviour to the species concerned (compare for example drinking and resting in lions; Veasey et al., 1996b). The reduction of aggression per se does not represent an improvement in animal welfare. However, if captive animals are expressing aggression at levels beyond what is normal for their wild conspecifics, then a reduction can be considered an animal-welfare improvement. Humans may not like to see aggression between animals but such aggressive behaviour can perform an important role in maintaining social order. In chimpanzees, for example, dominant males will usually support weaker individuals in aggressive encounters, thereby discouraging aggression within their social group. To support strong individuals would be to reward and thus increase the levels of aggression (Goodall, 1986).

The captive environment often exposes animals to a wide range of stressors, such as being handled by the animal care-giver, and these stressors can cause impairment of cognitive functions, e.g. memory. Most animals in captivity need to use cognitive functions such as memory to locate resources (e.g. food) within their environment. Thus, protecting cognitive functioning is an important aspect of environmental enrichment. The idea that increasing behavioural diversity improves animal welfare links to the idea that animals expressing a full range of wild behaviour patterns are experiencing an optimal level of welfare (see Veasey et al., 1996b). Previously, we have seen that this is not a strong measure of animal welfare. In zoos, however, the promotion of behavioural diversity might be of considerable importance in their conservation and education programmes (Kreger et al., 1998).

The costs of building an animal enclosure are, usually, directly proportional to the size of the enclosure (i.e. bigger equals more expensive) and space, therefore, should be fully utilised. However, does it matter to the animal that it does not utilise all the space in its enclosure or that it only spends short periods of time in certain areas? The answer depends on the reasons why the animal uses enclosure space as it does. Think about your own home: you spend most time in the bedroom, followed by the living-room, then the kitchen and finally the bathroom; the uses of these rooms reflects the principal behaviours expressed there, i.e. sleeping, socialising, cooking and comfort behaviours. The amount of time spent in a room does not reflect its importance – imagine a house without a bathroom. Stolba and Wood-Gush (1984) showed that given the opportunity, domestic pigs also will arrange their space into areas with different functions. Thus, in a well-designed environment we do not expect to see that animals use all areas equally but we do expect that they will use all areas. However, in a badly designed environment, animals may only use a limited amount of the space available due to lack of utilisable space. At Edinburgh Zoo (UK) it was noticed that the Bennett's wallabies only used the central area of their circular enclosure as they preferred to be as far away from zoo visitors as possible. The enclosure was modified by planting small bushy trees, which provided camouflage, along the enclosures perimeter; the wallabies then started to use nearly all the space in the enclosure. Thus, it is not space provision *per se* that is important but how the space is used in relation to the opportunities it provides for captive animals.

The promotion of 'desirable' behaviour patterns is immensely difficult to assess in terms of animal welfare, usually because the behaviour patterns deemed desirable for an animal to express are determined by humans not the animal. Chamove and Anderson (1989) have suggested the following four criteria to determine whether a behaviour pattern is desirable:

(1) normality – the behaviour approximates to that expressed in the wild;
(2) public acceptability – the public do not like to see abnormal behaviour, for example;
(3) theoretical considerations – the promotion of exercise based on wild time-budgets;
(4) practical considerations – reducing food wastage, for example.

However, the increase or decrease of many behaviour patterns are highly ambiguous in animal-welfare terms. Firstly, in the wild the duration of behaviour patterns is usually a function of resource availability and distribution (Veasey *et al.*, 1996b). Secondly, a large deviation from the duration expressed in the wild may reflect an improvement in animal welfare; captive giraffe, for example, spend much less time looking for predators than their wild counterparts, arguably an improvement in animal welfare (Veasey *et al.*, 1996a). Thirdly, the enrichment augmented expression of a behaviour pattern may have long-term negative consequences for animal welfare. Lemon and Barth (1992) found that increasing the feeding time, reduced longevity and adversely affected lifetime reproduction variables in zebra finches, e.g. weight of hatching chick. Thus, the promotion of certain behaviour patterns within the range expressed by wild conspecifics might improve animal welfare if they result from the provision of enrichment that allows animals to express motivation, i.e. behavioural needs (see above and Chapter 4; Hughes and Duncan, 1988).

Sambrook and Buchanan-Smith (1997) consider control over the environment to be *the* thing that results in environmental enrichment improving animal welfare. By control over the environment we mean that when the animal directs a motivated behaviour towards the environment, the environment provides opportunity for this behavioural expression and ultimately negative feedback that terminates this behaviour. Wild animals control their environment by expressing behaviour, the expression of foraging behaviour by a canary increases the probability that the animal will find food [obviously this is similar to Hughes and Duncan's (1988) concept of behavioural needs]. Thus, canaries control access to food through behavioural expression. In the scientific literature there has been considerable argument about the pros and cons of highly predictable and unpredictable environments (reviewed by Young, 1993). Those in favour of predictable environments cite evidence showing that predictable electric shocks for animals are less stressful than unpredictable shocks and therefore argue that animals can learn to adapt to a routine. Conversely those in favour of unpredictable environments point out that most animals evolved in unpredictable environments and that highly predictable environments are associated with the performance of abnormal behaviour (e.g. Lyons *et al.*, 1997). However, I feel that both sides are failing to understand what the expression of animal behaviour results in – it results in a greater probability that the animal will obtain its goal, i.e. it reduces unpredictability.

It has been demonstrated that control over the environment reduces emotionality in laboratory rats (Joffe *et al.*, 1973). In their experiment, rats could press levers (i.e. express control) to obtain water, food and light. The enclosures of these rats were yoked to control rats who received the same reward at the same time as the yoked operational rats. Mineka *et al.* (1986) conducted similar experiments with infant rhesus macaques and found a decrease in fear and increase in the coping responses of the individuals that could control their environment. In human children, there is evidence that control over their environment, or perception of control, has strong effects on their emotional, social and cognitive functioning (Gunnar, 1980). It is thought that this control may help prevent the onset of behavioural conditions such as learned helplessness, i.e. animals become withdrawn and inactive (Seligman, 1975). It should be noted that control over the environment is often associated with control over aversive events, e.g. the onset of an electric shock, but it also relates to control over positive events, e.g. access to a foraging enrichment device, (Young, 1993). Thus, it seems reasonable to accept that providing animals with control over their environment will improve animal welfare.

Learning ability allows an animal to cope with the changes in its environment. In a laboratory, the animal might be exposed to a new procedure, e.g. having blood withdrawn from its ear instead of its leg. The ability of the animal to learn what happens during this procedure, it has to move into a crush-cage, for example, will help it adapt to the change. On a farm, if cattle can learn the way to the milking parlour without being herded by a stockhand, the procedure will be less stressful. In the zoo, if animals learn that the rattling of keys means the keeper wishes the animal to go inside, this will be less stressful than being forced inside. A pet dog that can learn to predict the behaviour of its owner may be able to avoid the owner when they are in a bad mood. Thus, maintaining or augmenting an animal's learning ability can result in significant improvements in animal welfare.

Despite all my reservations and the comments expressed above, I believe the behavioural evidence overwhelmingly supports the hypothesis that environmental enrichment improves animal welfare.

3.1.2 Physiological evidence

The physiological evidence that environmental enrichment improves animal welfare is summarised in Table 3.2. In this table I have only included experimental studies that have been published in peer-reviewed journals. In many cases the enrichment study improved several aspects of animal welfare. I have explicitly excluded studies that only consider the usage of an enrichment device or technique.

Initially, physiological data are more appealing scientifically than behavioural evidence because they are so much easier to quantify – a hormone concentration is an exact physical quantity (e.g. $\mu l/ml$). This property of physiological data does not, however, make it a more reliable measure of animal welfare (see Terlouw *et al.*, 1997). The problem with much of the physiological evidence supporting the hypothesis that environmental enrichment improves animal welfare is that such data are usually generated by comparing barren to enriched environments. Often we do not have any data on the normal levels for a particular species; for example, we do not have baseline levels of circulating cortisol concentrations in wild animals. Thus, we cannot determine if enrichment merely returns levels to normal or actually enhances the situation in comparison to normal. However, we can determine whether enrichment improves animal welfare relatively, i.e. welfare in barren v. enriched environments. The remaining problem we have to assess is how reliable these measures are of animal welfare.

The use and validity of physiological measures of animal welfare has been reviewed by Terlouw *et al.*, (1997), therefore, I will only summarise the arguments. In Table 3.2, the most common physiological evidence was a reduction in cortisol level. Briefly, cortisol is produced in response to stressors, e.g. in the wild a predator, or in captivity being physically restrained, and it acts by stimulating the liver to rapidly release its energy reserves (Broom & Johnston, 1993). It is a measure that has been widely used in animal welfare research probably because it is simple to collect and assay from blood, urine or faeces. Undoubtedly, cortisol levels increase in response to stressors but they also increase in response to activity, feeding and excitement. Thus, the precise conditions of the experiments determine whether the change (reduction) in cortisol levels represents an improvement in animal welfare. For example, Beattie *et al.*, (2000a) found that pigs from enriched environments had higher cortisol levels but this was due to their greater activity levels not worse animal welfare. In response to environmental enrichment, improved immune system responses and decreases in physical conditions, such as stomach ulcerations, are unquestionably evidence of improvement in physical well-being and hence, animal welfare. However, as with cortisol, the experimen-

Table 3.2 The physiological evidence that environmental enrichment improves animal welfare.

Measure of improvement	Species	References
Reduction in plasma cortisol levels, including changes in adrenal size.	Mice, pigs, capuchins, rhesus macaques, leopard cats, blue fox (adults & cubs), horses.	Roy et al., 2001; Beattie et al., 2000a; de Groot et al., 2000; de Jong et al., 2000a; Boinski et al., 1999a; Boinski et al., 1999b; Schapiro et al., 1993; Carlstead et al., 1993; Ahola et al., 2000; McGreevy & Nicol, 1998; Pedersen, 1996.
Reduced stomach ulceration.	Rats.	Pare & Kluczynski, 1997.
Increase in noradrenaline levels.	Mice.	Naka et al., 2002.
Increased immune response, including ability to fight disease.	Mice, rhesus macaques, hamsters, long-tailed macaques, pigs.	Kingston & Hoffman-Goetz, 1996; Schapiro et al., 2000; Kuhnen, 1999; Capitanio & Lerche, 1998; Kelly et al., 2000.
Increased body weight from same food consumption.	Mice, goats, rhesus macaques.	Manosevitz & Joel, 1973; Manosevitz & Pryor, 1975; Van de Weerd et al., 1997; Flint & Murray, 2001; Schapiro & Kessel, 1993.
Facilitation of adolescent development.	Gerbils.	Cheal et al., 1986.
Changes in blood cell parameters.	Veal calves.	Wilson et al., 1999.

tal conditions under which the improvements occur are critical in assessing whether animal welfare has been improved. The response of other hormones and blood variables are reported (Table 3.2) to be evidence of improved animal welfare; again, these can be good measures of animal welfare but experimental details are critical.

The final improvement reported, the increase in body weight without increase in food consumption, relates to physical well-being. It suggests, that the animal's biological functioning has improved (Duncan & Fraser, 1997). Many other physiological measures of animal welfare exist, including: heart rate, heart-rate variability, blood pressure and other hormonal assays, e.g. prolactin. These tend to be less commonly used because of the difficulty in implementing them, and their interpretation in relation to animal welfare is experimental-situation-dependent.

3.1.3 Neurological evidence

The neurological evidence that environmental enrichment improves animal welfare is summarised in Table 3.3. In this table I have only included experimental studies that have been published in peer-reviewed journals. In many cases the enrichment study improved several aspects of animal welfare. I have explicitly excluded studies that only consider the usage of an enrichment device or technique.

Neurological data like physiological data can often be physically quantified and likewise appear to be reliable. Also, as with physiological data, we are usually comparing barren- and enriched-housed animals (except in the cases of induced brain damage). Psychologists have long been interested in the effects of environmental enrichment because it appears to speed-up or facilitate the repair of brain damage and often results in the improvement of cognitive or motor functions (Table 3.3). It has also been found that environmental enrichment can protect against cognitive deterioration that results from stressors or simply from ageing. Furthermore, there is evidence that it can improve cognitive functioning in animals, especially in the area of spatial information processing and memory (for a review see Healy & Tovée, 1999; Table 3.3). Thus, environmental enrichment indisputably improves cognitive functioning of animals. The proper cognitive functioning of an animal is vital for it to be able to adapt to changes in its environment (see 3.1.1 above for a discussion) and, therefore, important to animal welfare. Unfortunately, the vast majority of our neurological evidence comes from only two closely related species, rats and mice, which may raise questions about the general applicability of this evidence. However, to obtain neurological evidence we usually need to sacrifice the animals and this is not acceptable in most cases.

3.1.4 Other evidence

There is considerable evidence in the veterinary literature that environmental enrichment can minimise the possibility of pathogen tranmission, improve physical health of animals, help with the diagnosis of certain health problems, reduce

Table 3.3 The neurological evidence that environmental enrichment improves animal welfare.

Measure of improvement	Species	References
Increased brain cell density.	Rats, mice.	Johansson & Belichenko, 2002; Iuvone et al., 1996; Foster & Dumas, 2001.
Speeds recovery from brain damage – cellular recovery.	Gerbils, rats, mice.	Farrell et al., 2001; Dahlqvist et al., 2000; Dahlqvist et al., 1999; Torasdotter et al., 1998; Hannigan et al., 1993; Gomez-Pinilla et al., 1998; Schrott et al., 1992.
Changes brain biochemistry to augment learning or cognition.	Mice, rats.	Tang et al., 2001; Williams et al., 2001; Duffy et al., 2001; Ickes et al., 2000; Olsson et al., 1995.
Increased brain plasticity.	Rats.	Pinaud et al., 2001; Cotman & Berchtold, 1998; Torasdotter et al., 1996; Rasmuson et al., 1998.
Recovery of cognitive function following brain damage or cerebral deterioration.	Rats.	Biernaskie & Corbett, 2001; Passineau et al., 2001; Soffie et al., 1999; Young et al., 1999; Fernandez-Teruel et al., 1997; Hamm et al., 1996.
Recovery of motor abilities following brain damage.	Rats.	Borlongan, 2000; Johansson, 1996.
Enhanced (non-spatial) memory.	Mice, rats.	Hoplight et al., 2001; Woodcock & Richardson, 2000; Gagne et al., 1998; Escorihuela et al., 1995.
Increased brain weight and size.	Rats.	Greer et al., 1981; Ferchmin et al., 1975.
Improved visual perception.	Mice.	Prusky et al., 2000.
Improved spatial memory.	Rats.	Tees, 1999b; Barnes & McNaughton, 1985; Blakemore & Mitchell, 1973.
Enhanced social and other forms of cognition.	Rats, owl monkeys, squirrel monkeys.	Pham et al., 1999a; Xerri et al., 1996.
Modification of brain emotional systems:	Rats.	Chapillon et al., 1999.

the incidence of bodily sores and reduce the incidence of oral and gingival health problems (Baer, 1998; Young, 1997). The value of this physical health evidence to animal-welfare improvements that can result from environmental enrichment are immense. However, rarely in behavioural or physiological studies of environmental enrichment are physical health data collected. Too often we have only anecdotal data, such as animal care-givers reporting that the animals are much more difficult to catch as a result of increased physical fitness. One notable exception to this trend were the experiments into the use of different floor substrates for primates, reported by Chamove and Anderson (1989) who collected both behavioural data and data on the possibility of pathogen transmission. Thus, it may be that many enrichment studies are resulting in physical benefits but these data are not being collected, so I would encourage researchers to collect these data.

In other evidence, there is only one study from many conducted that shows environmental enrichment improves meat quality (Klont *et al.*, 2001). It seems, therefore, that the evidence for this improvement is weak. Kreger *et al.* (1998) discuss at length how environmental enrichment enhances the goals of the modern zoo by making animals behave normally, thus enhancing their education, conservation, research and recreation value. Finally, it has been demonstrated that foraging enrichment can help prevent animals from destroying the plants and structure of their enclosure (Embury, 1997).

3.2 How does Enrichment Improve Animal Welfare?

Tables 3.1 to 3.3 and the other evidence presented above show that there are many ways in which environmental enrichment can improve animal welfare. Many of these ways are highly interconnected. Often we do not understand the interconnections because studies have not attempted to measure all types of evidence and how they co-vary. Disentangling what has actually caused the improvement in animal welfare is a complex task, which I will illustrate by way of example. An increase in learning ability has often been reported as a result of environmental enrichment (Table 3.1). This improvement in learning ability will have a neurological basis, such as increased brain cell density (Table 3.2). A behavioural consequence of increased learning ability could be that animals are able to learn that humans are not a source of aversive experience. Thus, the animals' levels of fear for humans may be reduced (Table 3.1) and this may be associated with the reduction in cortisol levels (Table 3.2). But what actually resulted in an improvement in animal welfare? In this case, the improvement in animal welfare has come from a reduction in fear.

Let us look at another example. In an enclosure for deer we plant many trees and bushes to provide cover and places to hide because we notice they perform abnormal behaviour when people stand close to their enclosure. We find that the enrichment results in a reduction in the performance of abnormal behaviour

(Table 3.1), a reduction in blood pressure and increase in spatial memory. But what actually resulted in an improvement in animal welfare? Here, I would argue that the deer's opportunity to express hiding behaviour, the opportunity to express control over its environment, has improved animal welfare.

One final example: for guinea pigs we enrich their enclosures by providing them with a range of toys that are changed on a daily basis. The guinea pigs respond to these toys by engaging in play behaviour and being less fearful when handled (Table 3.1). The measurement of their heart rate when handled now shows no significant increases. Investigations into their spatial memory demonstrates an enhancement (Table 3.3). But what actually resulted in an improvement in animal welfare? The toys have acted as a visually novel stimulus and this has caused the increase in spatial memory but it is the exposure to novelty that has reduced the actual levels of fear (Table 3.1) and improved welfare.

Thus, the provision of behavioural opportunities (or if you prefer 'empowerment') to allow an animal to express control over its environment or the provision of stimuli (e.g. novel objects) that result in fear reduction are, I believe, the mechanisms underlying how environmental enrichment improves animal welfare. One other possibility I have not discussed because of the lack of experimental evidence is that enrichment is intrinsically rewarding to the animal, i.e. the animal-welfare benefits are accrued from the 'enjoyment' the animal receives. The evidence that animals choose to use a puzzle feeder when food is freely available in a bowl (i.e. contra-freeloading), for example, relates to information gathering behaviour rather than hedonistic behaviour (see Chapter 4; Inglis *et al.*, 1997). Perhaps subjective approaches to the study of animal welfare, such as those proposed by Wemelsfelder *et al.* (Wemelsfelder & Lawrence, 2001; Wemelsfelder *et al.*, 2001; Wemelsfelder, 2001; Wemelsfelder *et al.*, 2000b; Wemelsfelder *et al.*, 2000a) may illuminate this approach.

Proactive v. Reactive use of Environmental Enrichment

In an ideal world, the captive environment of a species would be designed with perfect knowledge of the species' requirements to experience an optimal level of animal welfare. The animal-management systems would also reflect this perfect knowledge. At the very least, animal enclosures and management systems should be designed with the most up-to-date and reliable information that exists in relation to animal welfare. Unfortunately, the latter case tends to be the exception rather than the rule. Usually, environmental enrichment is an afterthought and is added in once the enclosure is built. This is the reality under which we often work. Most commercial animal housing tends to be used until the buildings fall down, except in the case of laboratories where changing regulations forces more frequent updating. (I remember one zoo director telling me that every animal enclosure should have a time bomb built into it which would destroy the building after 25 years!) Some of the buildings in the world's older zoos, London, for example, are more than a hundred years old (Bostock, 1993; Krohn *et al.*, 1999). Many old buildings are protected by law as architectural heritage that cannot be significantly altered and some institutions are forced to continue using them due to lack of land for expansion. This is a common problem for the older zoos within the UK (where architectural conservation can be impinging on species conservation). Thus, many buildings were constructed before the concept of animal welfare had even appeared within the scientific community's consciousness. Unfortunately, it is in these types of buildings that people mostly have to work with environmental enrichment, that is, starting with a poorly designed building. Starting from a poor base always makes the implementation of improvements difficult.

4.1 What Animals Want

Environmental enrichment is largely about providing the animal with opportunities to express behaviour patterns for which it is highly motivated. In the past, there was a tendency for animal welfare scientists to measure what caused animal-welfare problems and to try and counter these problems – a reactive approach. This should not surprise us given that in any problem solving situation, the first step is to recognise that a problem exists and then to quantify the problem. Unfortunately, in my opinion far too much time, effort and money has gone into quantifying animal problems and not enough into solutions. For example, the textbook on animal welfare by Appleby and Hughes (1997) contains eleven chapters associated with problems and their assessment and only four chapters on solutions. Imagine the public outcry if such an imbalance existed in the field of human medicine. I am certainly not denying the importance of assessing welfare problems and obtaining solid scientific information to understand them, but merely suggesting we need more solutions. I suspect that part of the problem lies in the fact that it is easier to quantify a problem, than to think of workable solutions.

The first scientific attempts to find out what animals wanted in their environment started with the Brambell Report (1965). One of the authors of this report on the effects of intensive farming on animal welfare in the UK, was the Oxford zoologist, Thorpe. Previous to his involvement in this report, Thorpe (Brambell, 1965) had noticed that relocated African buffalo preferred their relocation pen to the wild environment because of the food, shelter and protection. Thorpe realised that the buffalo were able to make a logical choice, and it was this observation that gave rise to the choice test. The choice testing of animals was a popular way to try and establish animal preferences throughout the 1970s and early 1980s. However, it was heavily criticised by Duncan (1978) who argued that animals in choice tests only chose the least aversive option. More recently, the choice test has been largely abandoned due to these theoretical objections, or it is used in very applied situations such as assessing the suitability of several competing products (e.g. Mills *et al.*, 2000; but for a review concerning choice tests see Fraser & Matthews, 1997).

In 1983, Marian Dawkins started to investigate what was important to domestic hens by applying consumer-demand theory (a branch of behavioural economics) to their behaviour. This work represented a major shift in the way that animal-welfare scientists were thinking. Rather than measuring the adverse effects of captivity on animal welfare, scientists now had a methodology to ask the animal what it wanted but without the theoretical objections that choice tests suffer. At the centre of this theory is that animals, when faced with a limited budget (the currency is usually energy or time), will behave like a logical human consumer. Human consumers buy fewer luxury products (e.g. ice cream) and maintain their consumption of essential products (e.g. bread) when the cost of these products increases and their income does not. Dawkins (1983) applied this theory to the choices made by domestic hens and found that they too act like logical consumers. For example, hens were prepared to pay much higher costs to obtain food than to obtain social companionship but would pay significant costs for social companionship. Thus, Dawkins initiated an animal-centred approach to animal welfare, one that had potential to be proactive rather than merely reactive. It was also an approach that allowed animals to rate the relative value of resources and was, therefore, attractive to animal welfare scientists working with farm animal species, since providing these animals with every need would be economically and practically unfeasible. Thus, the method provided a way of prioritising animal needs.

The application of consumer-demand theory (behavioural economics) has been a productive area of animal welfare research during the 1990s (for a review see Young, 1999). However, the interpretation of these experiments has been widely debated in the scientific journals (Ng, 1995; Mason *et al.*, 1998). In 2001 Mason *et al.* published a groundbreaking experiment on the use of behavioural-economic theory to analyse what is important to farmed mink. In their experiment, mink were housed in a closed-economy experimental cage that contained seven chambers that the mink could enter by pushing open weighted one-way doors. The weight on the doors could be increased and inside each chamber was a resource, such as a novel object, a toy, a swimming pool, the opportunity to see another mink, an empty chamber etc. By increasing the weight on the doors, Mason *et al.* (2001) were able to determine which resources were most important to the mink. The results showed that mink quickly stopped visiting the room with the toy but continued to visit the swimming pool even when the weight used was more than their body weight. Mason *et al.* then looked at depriving the mink of the swimming pool; cortisol assays (a hormonal measurement of stress) revealed that swimming pool deprivation was as stressful to the mink as food deprivation.

The work of Dawkins (1983), and Mason *et al.* (2001) has provided a proactive way for assessing the welfare requirements of animals. Young (1999) has suggested that behavioural resilience could be used to assess the welfare needs of animals in captive environments. The behavioural resilience of an animal is how the animal responds to having less time to perform its daily time budget. For example, if we force an animal to spend more time foraging by scattering its food around its enclosure, which behaviours decrease in their duration and which remain at their normal level? The assumption being that the more important behaviours will remain at their normal level of daily time-budget expression. Young (1999) suggested that such an experimental situation could be induced in any animal's enclosure by mixing its food with inert substrates, forcing it to spend more time foraging, and analysing the subsequent changes in its time budget.

A cautionary note about the use of behavioural economics, is that it tends to make us focus on what things are essential for animal well-being. Hughes and Duncan (1988) noted that the problem for captive animals is that they have lots of time and nothing to do. Therefore, they suggest, somewhat paradoxically, that in this situation luxury behaviours fulfil a vital role in occupying the animals' time budget. Normally, we provide captive animals with all of their requirements for physical well-being, and so it is the luxuries that are usually missing from their existence. Inglis *et al.* (2001) has suggested that when captive animals have all of their physiological requirements met, they then switch to information gathering behaviour – or exploratory behaviour (Inglis *et al.*, 1997; Inglis *et al.*, 2001).

Clearly, behavioural-economic analysis of animal behaviour has a role to play in identifying essential and luxury behaviour patterns. The necessity of such behaviour patterns for animal welfare depends on the resources within the animal's environment and how it is being managed. Breeding sows are kept in a permanent state of hunger, due to economic and fertility reasons, whereas red river hogs housed in a zoo have all of their physiological needs provided for. In the case of the breeding sow, she is motivated to express foraging behaviour to find food, i.e. an essential behaviour that restores physiological processes (Young, 1993). The red river hog, instead, is motivated to gather information about its environment, i.e. a luxury behaviour that is non-physiologically restorative. Conceivably, the enrichment solution to both animals' behavioural need (see Hughes & Duncan, 1988) is to cover the floor of the enclosure in forest-bark chippings and scatter the animals' food into it. The behaviour expressed by our two species may look the same to us human observers but may have different significance for the species concerned. In general, for companion, laboratory and zoo animals, human care-givers provide all their physiological needs; hence, the expression of luxury behaviours are more important. Farm animals tend to be much more restricted and the expression of essential behaviours is more important (Hughes & Duncan, 1988).

4.2 Prioritising Environmental Enrichment

How do we prioritise which species to enrich first? There is no simple answer to this question. Arguably, one could use a species' potential to suffer as a prioritising tool but how do we define a species' potential to suffer? One possibility is to examine the cognitive abilities of species, since suffering can be regarded as a mental state. Byrne (1999) took exactly this approach and reviewed the primate cognition literature to determine which species are most likely to suffer from exposure to barren environments. In his review of the literature Byrne considered the ability to predict future circumstances as critical in the assessment of a species' ability to suffer. He concluded that only chimpanzees deserved special consideration based on cognition experiments, although he did of course recognise that all species have the capacity to suffer. I think his definition of capacity to suffer is too limited; as Jeremy Bentham pointed out: 'The question is not, can they reason? Nor can they talk, but can they suffer?' (see Chapter 1). Byrne's proposal produces only a two-point scale, humans/chimpanzees and the rest of the Animal Kingdom, which is not very useful for our purposes. In addition, outside of primates, rodents and parrots, the cognitive abilities of relatively few species have been investigated. So does any kind of universal measure of animal cognitive abilities exist? We cannot use brain size as this is merely a correlate of body size. Some researchers in the past tried to use encephalisation quotient, the ratio of brain to body weight, which should remove the body weight–brain size correlation. However, the brains of animals are not uniform structures, they do not operate like a central processing unit (CPU), different areas of the brain control different abilities or functions. In general, we can divide the animal brain into those areas that control bodily functions (such as respiration) and those associated with cognitive processes. The ratio of these two areas is known as the neocortex ratio (Aiello & Dunbar, 1993; Dunbar, 1992, 1995, 1998; Pawlowski et al., 1998). It is possible to calculate the neocortex volume of mammalian brains if we have the species brain volume (Dunbar & Bever, 1998). Numerous research studies have found that species with high neocortex ratios (e.g. chimpanzees and dolphins) perform extremely well in tests of animal cognition (Byrne, 2000; Pawlowski et al., 1998; Dunbar, 1998) and display the highest levels of spontaneously occurring cognitive problem solving, e.g. tactical deception (Byrne & Whiten, 1988). Such species also tend to live in large complex social groups (Dunbar, 1992, 1995, 1998; Dunbar & Bever, 1998). I am suggesting in situations where we have to prioritise our implementation of environmental enrichment, due to lack of resources such as time and money, then neocortex ratio would be one non-arbitrary measure we could use. The use of this measurement is likely to prove popular with the public as popular species such as primates and cetaceans top this scale. What I am suggesting is of course highly specist (see Ryder, 1989) but I am not suggesting that species with low neocortex ratios cannot suffer, just that perhaps they have less capacity to suffer. The use of this scale as a measure of capacity to suffer also strongly correlates with the approach of Byrne (1999). A number of animal welfare scientists have defined animal welfare as being about how an animal feels about its world (Duncan, 1996; Dawkins, 1990); that is, animal welfare as a mental state.

The proposed use of neocortex ratio should work relatively well for mammals, where much data has been published on brain volume (a number of databases exist on the internet). For other groups such as birds, reptiles, fish and amphibians, the significance of neocortex ratio is not understood. The suggestion I make is that we use correlates of high levels of cognition and neocortex ratio. The easiest correlate to use of these two related factors is social-group size and social complexity. For example, within the birds, parrots live in large flocks and form long-term stable social bonds e.g. most parrot species are life-long monogamists. Research on parrot cognition by Pepperberg (1998, 1994, 1993a, 1993b, 1983; Pepperberg & Funk, 1990; Pepperberg et al., 2000) strongly supports the idea that they possess advanced cognition abilities. Therefore, we should accord a high priority to this family within the bird class.

Once we move outside the mammal and bird classes it is difficult to use such cognitive scales. I have heard some scientists express the opinion that reptiles, amphibians and fish have minimal behavioural needs and therefore their requirements for a good level of animal welfare are lower (e.g. Poole, 1992). These scientists, however, are failing to give these species the benefit of the doubt, we simply do not have the scientific evidence to know if they can suffer like mammals and birds. Sometimes, as in the case of the octopus, we have cognition experiments (Mather, 1995) that can guide our considerations. In other cases perhaps we have nothing more to rely on than the casual observations of animal care-givers, and their associated beliefs. In aquariums many animal care-givers report that sharks, for example, appear to swim stereotypically but they may just be performing patrolling behaviour in a limited environment. The expression of abnormal behaviour may be of some use in identifying species that we should prioritise for environmental enrichment but abnormal behaviour is not an unambiguous or the only indicator of welfare problems (Mason, 1991). If you were to ask zoo keepers which species performed the most abnormal behaviour they would probably answer the lions, and studies of big cats confirm this to be the case (see Lyons et al., 1997). This is an interesting observation because lions have the second highest neocortex ratio of any carnivore species (Dunbar & Bever, 1998), they live in complex social groups (Grinnell & McComb, 1996) and appear to have highly developed social cognitive abilities (McComb et al., 1994; Grinnell & McComb, 2001).

Maple and Perkins (1996) have also considered using comparative psychology to provide information about the prioritising of species for enrichment. In addition, they suggest we could use species' inherent levels of curiosity or exploration as a measure to divide species into categories for prioritisation. Interestingly, they also suggest the use of ecological data; they note that omnivores and opportunists demonstrate the most exploratory and inquisitive behaviour.

Finally, Ros Clubb and Georgia Mason (1998) at the University of Oxford, UK have been investigating life-history (e.g. age at sexual maturity) and behavioural characteristics (e.g. home-range size) that might be predictors of a carnivore species' propensity to develop abnormal behaviour in captivity. These researchers began by surveying all the literature and unpublished reports (e.g. undergraduate and postgraduate student theses) on the incidence of abnormal behaviour in carnivores housed in UK zoos and then looked for relationships between life-history or behavioural characteristics and the level of abnormal behaviour expressed. Thus, their study was a meta-analysis of existing data. The results show that the best predictor of the propensity of a carnivore species to develop abnormal behaviour in captivity is home-range size. The further a species travels each day when hunting the greater the probability that it will develop abnormal behaviour when it is maintained in captivity. Perhaps this also suggests that an outlet for hunting motivation is very important in such species (see Williams et al., 1996). As a minimum we now know which species require greater attention to their housing requirements before we place them in captivity. Meta-analyses, such as this, on other groups' and classes' propensity to develop abnormal behaviour may in the future provide us with a useful tool to prioritise species for environmental enrichment. Of course, this also depends on the fact that abnormal behaviour will continue to be accepted as a reliable animal welfare indicator (see Chapter 3; Mason, 1991).

From the above information we can construct the following selection rules for prioritising environmental enrichment:

- Does the species have the ability to predict future events?
- Do cognition experiments support the proposition that the species functions at a high cognitive level?
- Does the species have a large neocortex ratio?
- Does the species live in large social groups with complex and long-lived interactions?
- Does the species demonstrate high levels of curiosity or exploratory behaviour?
- Is the species known to usually display abnormal behaviour in captivity?
- Is the species opportunist or omnivore?

The judicious use of the above selection rules is a start towards developing a system for prioritising the implementation of environmental enrichment for captive animals. I have put the rules in order of what I consider to be most important using empirical observations, but the prioritising of these rules is subjective. The use of subjective information is both controversial and interesting: controversial because it does not follow the scientific method, and interesting because of the results it generates. Wemelsfelder *et al.* (2001) have demonstrated that naive human observers can accurately identify and describe functional differences between pigs that have been reared in barren or enriched environments. In their experiments, the pigs are presented 'blind' to the observers in a neutral arena. Thus, these experiments point to the intriguing possibility in the future of using human subjective assessments of animal welfare. Perhaps in the future human subjective assessment could be added to the list of prioritising rules mentioned above.

4.3 Solving Animal-welfare Problems using Environmental Enrichment

In the previous sections I have dealt with the ideal world of proactive environmental enrichment strategies. Despite the well known fact that it is easier to prevent a (welfare) problem than cure it, many institutions are reactive to animal-welfare problems. Unfortunately, the great motivator for many institutions to implement environmental enrichment is when an animal-welfare problem appears. Normally, the motivator is the appearance of a locomotor stereotypy (e.g., repetitive route tracing) or self-injurious behaviour (e.g., fur plucking), i.e. gross and visually obvious problems but I am concerned than many non-visually obvious welfare problems are missed. The common response of institutions to such problems is to either block the behaviour (e.g. place objects along a pacing animal's chosen pacing route) or to provide many different kinds of environmental enrichment. Often, such solutions do not improve the animal's welfare, although they may remove the visual indicators of the welfare problem, since our pacing animal can no longer pace, for example.

Although when we discover an animal welfare problem our goal is to solve the problem, this can only be done by first assessing the problem. First of all, does a real welfare problem exist or is it just a perceived problem? Lions sleep for 20 hours per day in zoo environments and the public often complain that this is evidence that they are bored. However, data on wild lions show that they also sleep 20 hours a day and forcing them to be more active would probably be detrimental to their welfare. Thus, we need a good understanding of all aspects of a species' life. If we decide a real welfare problem exists our next step must be to assess the problem. Suppose our welfare problem is a pet dog that pulls out its fur. What we need is a full description of its environment and the circumstances under which this behaviour is occurring. We may well discover that the dog is left alone in its owner's house for nine hours each day while the owner is out at work. Furthermore, that it is only during this time, when the dog is left alone, that it pulls out its fur (the dog has never been seen to perform this behaviour in front of the owner). Thus, we now have a suggestion of causation, the problem may be caused by prolonged social isolation each day. We can now select appropriate enrichment strategies that might include: the owner changing their work schedule to spend more time with the dog; the owner hiring someone to walk the dog while they are at work; the owner buying another dog to provide company for the existing dog; or the owner placing the dog with people that have more time to interact socially with it.

My experience suggests that the sooner the problem is addressed the more likely it is that environmental enrichment will be effective in treating the problem. Unfortunately, once certain kinds of welfare problems have been established in an animal's behaviour repertoire they become irreversible. In zoos there are many cases of carnivores that have been moved from a barren zoo, where they developed abnormal behaviour, to a new zoo where, despite huge amounts of prolonged efforts to enrich the animals' lives, the abnormal behaviour continues in the exact same form and pattern. Abnormal behaviour such as stereotypies can become emancipated from their original causation (Mason, 1991). It is vital, therefore, to treat animal-welfare problems while the original cause is still the source of the problem. Cooper and Nicol (1991) found that bank voles with established abnormal behaviour (abnormally repetitive somersaulting) preferred barren to enriched environments as these environments facilitated the performance of the abnormal behaviour (easier to somersault in an open space). Clearly, once an animal is in this state it will be much more difficult to treat.

Returning to our 'lonely' dog example – too often, the owner does not consider causation and focuses only on the effects of the behaviour, i.e. the dog pulling out fur. So the owner provides a substitute for the dog to pull fur from, a rabbit skin, for example, but of course this does not work because the animal is motivated to perform self-directed behaviour not fur pulling *per se*. In desperation, the owner may take the dog to a veterinary surgeon who prescribes either some tranquillisers, which eliminate the undesired behaviour, or a Victorian collar, which blocks the behaviour. Hopefully, you can see that these latter solutions only either hide the welfare problem – the tranquillisers, or treat the symptoms – the Victorian collar: neither of which improves the animal's welfare (see Chapter 3). While on the subject of the use of drugs to solve animal-welfare problems, I am not against the use of drugs *per se* but the type of drugs used should be those that facilitate the resolution of the animal-welfare problem.

4.4 Summary: Treating Welfare Problems

To summarise, when you have a welfare problem that you think can be treated by environmental enrichment, then you should follow these steps:

* identify the problem;
* assess the problem;
* identify probable causation;
* treat the cause of the problem;
* assess the effectiveness of the solution;

In our fur-pulling dog example it would always be wise to get a veterinary surgeon's opinion on the problem as it may have an organic cause. For example, I know of one case where a pet dog suddenly started to become aggressive when anyone approached him. To an animal behaviourist a logical explanation is that the animal has had an experience that makes it associate people with physical threats. However, the veterinary surgeon quickly found the problem; the dog was going blind and could no longer visually recognise anyone.

I would like to finish this chapter with a plea: please, please be proactive in your use of environmental enrichment and knowledge concerning animal welfare.

Designing an Enrichment Device

5.1 Identifying What You Want to Do

It might sound a little obvious, but before you design an environmental enrichment device you need to know what you want it to do. The goal of an enrichment device should relate to the goals of environmental enrichment as outlined in Chapter 1. Examples of potential goals include the promotion of foraging behaviour to create a wild-type time budget. However, much more useful is to think of the form of the foraging behaviour, e.g. hunting, ambushing, browsing, grazing, etc. (see Chapter 8). The application of environmental enrichment should never be on the basis of trying anything just in case it improves animal welfare, such an approach will be more likely to decrease animal welfare.

5.1.1 Sources of inspiration

The sources of inspiration for an environmental enrichment device should come from a clear understanding of why you are designing the device (see examples in the next section). Only then can we apply creative processes, such as brain storming, which usually works best with a group of people, i.e. the enrichment circle (see Chapter 6). For example, I have always looked for help and advice from mechanical engineers in the design of enrichment devices. Usually, I have found such expertise in the local university. All ideas should be written down, presented to the group and the pros and cons discussed. It is also extremely useful to consider similar enrichment devices that may already exist as sources of inspiration.

5.2 Importance of Species-specific Behaviour

Once we have a goal or target behaviour we wish to enrich, then we need to have a detailed understanding of this behaviour in the species concerned. I will illustrate this by way of two examples, the extractive foraging behaviour of pigs and the hunting (chases) of cheetah. The behaviour of each species has been shaped by the processes of evolution so that the species concerned can fill a particular ecological niche. Thus, to a lesser or greater extent all behaviour is species-specific. It is important to have a full understanding of the situation under which the animal lives as well as the species-specific behaviour you wish to enrich. Failure to provide an appropriate outlet for species-specific behaviour can mean that the animal is unable to obtain the reinforcement on offer due to the incompatibility between the reward and the behaviour required to obtain it (Young *et al.*, 1994a). However, as Young (1997) notes, more cognitively complex animals are often more able to learn non-species-specific behaviours.

Female breeding pigs (sows) are food restricted for economic and reproductive reasons. This food restriction causes a higher level of hunger and to fulfil this motivation pigs normally express foraging behaviour (appetitive behaviour) to find food and then feed (consummatory behaviour). In the wild, pigs are extractive foragers, which means they usually find small but variable quantities of nutrient-dense food that is dispersed relatively randomly in space. The occurrence of food is also not predictable in time. Foraging behaviour of pigs is characterised by rooting behaviour (the turning over of natural substrates with the snout), walking and sniffing to locate the presence of food (pigs do not possess high levels of visual acuity). I took this information and used it to develop design criteria for a foraging device for domestic sows (see Young, 1997):

- The device would facilitate the expression of species-specific foraging behaviour by allowing this behaviour to be directed towards it, i.e. rooting, walking and sniffing.
- In response to species-specific behaviour directed towards the device, the device would deliver an appropriate food reward.
- The reward would be delivered randomly within the space of the animals' enclosure.
- The timing of the food reward deliveries would be a random interval between successive rewards, such that the animal could not predict when it would receive a food reward.
- The amount of food that the animal received during each reward would be a random amount with a minimum that is sufficient to maintain foraging behaviour, e.g. 30 g for domestic sows.
- The device should have no moving parts to ensure that the probabilities of breakdown were minimal.
- The device should require no electronic parts and, therefore, no power sources to ensure the minimum of maintenance and minimal possibilities that it would breakdown.
- The device should be easy to clean and quick to fill as on farms the stockhands' time is extremely valuable.

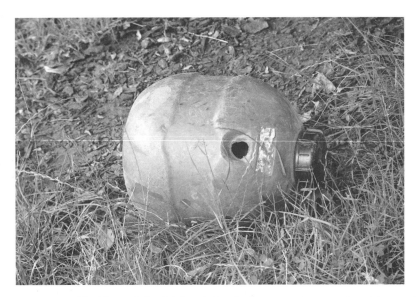

Figure 5.1 A modified form of the Edinburgh Foodball – an environmental enrichment device for use with hoof-stock – © Robert J. Young (see Young *et al.*, 1994).

- The device should pose no safety risks to the target animals, e.g. the domesticated sows.

The expression of the species-specific foraging behaviour was facilitated by designing the device to be a large sphere (Figure 5.1). The curvature of the sphere permitted the pig to place its snout under the ball and then lift its snout as if it was turning over substrate i.e. 'rooting'. This action cause the sphere to roll forward. (We noticed that when the pig performed the root with its snout it also made an audible sniff, which is what pigs do in the wild when foraging.) Inside the sphere was a mechanism that dispensed food to the inside of the sphere in response to being rooted. The sphere itself had one small food dispensing hole and it was only when this hole touched the ground that food was dispensed to the pig. Thus, food was dispensed in different places in the pigs' enclosure in respond to species-specific foraging behaviour. However, the amount of food dispensed was dependent on the number of times the food dispensing mechanism was operated (dependent on how the foraging device was rooted) and delivered food to the inside of the sphere before being released through the food dispensing hole. The timing between food deliveries was dependent upon when the food dispensing hole made contact with the ground. Thus, these features recreate the implementation of species-specific behaviour and natural patterns of reinforcement. In terms of practicalities, the sphere was made of fibreglass which facilitated rapid cleaning (with a pressure hose); the device had a quick fill mechanism for the internal food dispensing mechanism; the fibreglass sphere was strong and relatively cheap to manufacture. Finally, the sphere was covered in 30 mm high pintles ('lumps') which prevented dirt or water entering the inside of the sphere and contaminating the food. Studies with the foraging device ('The Edinburgh Foodball') demonstrated its value in allowing the expression of motivated foraging and the creation of wild-type time budgets for domestic sows (Young & Lawrence, 1996; Young *et al.*, 1994).

In zoos, cheetahs rarely express hunting behaviour because they are not provided with the opportunity to do so. It is thought that this lack of expression of hunting behaviour may cause the expression of abnormal behaviour and physical health problems (Williams *et al.*, 1996). In the wild, cheetahs hunt by chasing their prey at high speed over short distances, normally less than 200 metres. The cheetah finds its prey by using its modified visual system (it has a row of densely packed cones running across the back of the retina). Once the prey is detected, the cheetah attempts to get as close as possible by stalking before it runs after the prey. The cheetah uses its speed to catch up with its prey and then it slows down. Prey are caught by being tripped, the cheetah striking at the legs of its prey with a forelimb. Once tripped, the cheetah kills the prey using a throat bite to strangle it. In the wild, cheetahs normally hunt successfully only once per day. I used this information to develop design criteria for a hunting enrichment device for captive cheetahs (see Young, 1997):

- It should stimulate species-specific hunting behaviour, i.e. short distance high speed chases.
- The cheetah should use its specialised visual system to detect its 'prey', i.e. a system designed to detect moving objects in the horizontal plane.
- The 'prey' should be pursued at high speed before it is caught or manages to escape.
- The cheetah should only have the opportunity to capture the 'prey' while it is moving at high speed through the enclosure.
- The method of capture used must be species-specific, i.e. the 'prey' is hit with the forelimb of the cheetah and this causes it to fall over.
- The availability of 'prey' should mimic that in the wild, in particular the cheetah should not control the availability of prey (see Synder, 1977).
- The device should be highly practical, i.e. minimum of moving parts, cheap to construct, easy to clean and quick to use.

The enrichment device essentially consisted of a wire running at 2 metres high for the whole length of the cheetahs' enclosure (Figure 5.2). Along the wire ran a pulley system from which was suspended a bait (usually a dead rabbit). The pulley system moved at high speed through the enclosure under the influence of gravity. The bait was held at 0.5 metres above the ground: it was not caught by

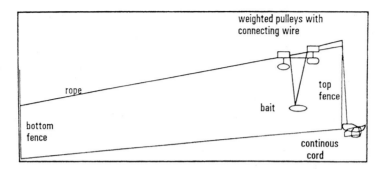

Figure 5.2   An engineer's drawing of a hunting enrichment device for captive cheetahs – © Robert J. Young (see Williams *et al.*, 1996).

the cheetah before the end of the run it was automatically lifted out of the chee-tahs' reach to prevent them waiting at the end of the run. Thus, in terms of behaviour, the bait was detected by its high speed horizontal movement, the cheetah had to chase the bait and catch it while it was moving. The number of runs was determined by the human operator who provided only enough runs for the cheetah to catch one bait per day. The system had few moving parts, required little maintenance, was easy to operate and cheap to construct (but it did require a sloping enclosure). The implementation of the device permitted cheetahs to express species-specific hunting behaviour and it augmented the cheetahs' interest in prey (the black buck it could see from its enclosure, for example).

To summarise, the key characteristics of any design criteria for environmental enrichment devices are:

(1)   The important components of the behaviour need to be identified and described to facilitate behavioural expression.
(2)   The reinforcement schedule should mimic that of the wild to prevent the development of behavioural problems.
(3)   How to implement the characteristics in points 1 and 2 needs considering. In addition, one should consider how the animal might try to 'beat the system'.
(4)   The practicalities of the system need serious consideration, i.e. cost, maintenance, cleaning, ease of use and probability of breaking down.

5.3 Rewards and Schedules of Reward

Anything that motivates an animal to perform a behaviour again can be considered to be a reward or reinforcer. When an animal expresses a behaviour pattern that is essential for survival, the performance of this behaviour is reinforced by the release of chemicals (e.g. opioids) within the brain. Reinforcers can be divided into primary reinforcers and secondary reinforcers. Primary reinforcers are those that directly reward the performance of a behaviour pattern, e.g. the food given to a dog when it performs a trick. Secondary reinforcers are stimuli associated with the presentation of a primary reinforcer, e.g. if a whistle is blown just before a dog is given a food reward, the dog will associate the whistle with food and the whistle will become a secondary reinforcer (Mellen & Ellis, 1996). Often, secondary reinforcers are used to provide additional reinforcement in animal training programmes (Desmond & Laule, 1994).

Psychologists recognise many different types of reward schedules. Principally, reward schedules vary in the time between reinforcers, the number of responses between reinforcers, and the amount of reinforcement received (Chance, 1998):

(1) How variable the schedule is in terms of time between consecutive rewards, e.g. fixed interval (once every 30 seconds) or variable interval (on average once every 30 seconds). This factor often relates to the spatial distribution of the reward in the wild.
(2) The variability of the appetitive behaviour the animal must express to obtain a reward, e.g. fixed schedule (after each five repetitions of the behaviour) or variable schedule (on average after five repetitions of the behaviour). This factor usually relates to the success rate of the behaviour in the wild.
(3) How variable the quantity of the reward is, e.g. fixed (30 g of food) or variable (on average 30 g of food). This relates to the reward size encountered in the wild.

5.3.1 Use of food rewards

The most common design fault involving environmental enrichment devices is for the device to dispense food unnecessarily. The only devices that should dispense food are those whose purpose are to stimulate feeding, foraging or hunting behaviour. Why not use devices with other goals, such as stimulating play behaviour, to dispense food? Any device that dispenses food will certainly prove to be highly attractive to animals that use it, since food acquisition behaviour is a highly motivated behaviour pattern that restores physiological homeostasis. Food is a great motivator as studies into animal learning and training demonstrate (Bloomsmith *et al.*, 1998; Mellen & Ellis, 1996; Desmond & Laule, 1994; Clark & Boyer, 1993; Askew, 1996), and its association with an enrichment device will almost certainly result in that device being used (O'Connor, 2000; Spring *et al.*, 1997; Holmes *et al.*, 1995). Human nature being what it is, the designer of an enrichment device wishes it to be a success and the measure of success is how much the device is used. Young & Lawrence (1996), for example, showed that a foraging device for pigs would be used for the majority of the pigs' waking hours.

As a hypothetical case, imagine we have designed an environmental-enrichment device the purpose of which is to facilitate play behaviour in pigs. Our device might essentially just be a ball with some material inside that makes a noise when the pigs play with the device. What would be the effect of making the device also dispense food on use of the device? The pigs would learn to associate use of the device with food. Once the device has dispensed all its food it would no longer be used by the pigs because the primary reinforcing property of the device was food. Young *et al.* (1996, 1994) found this to be the case for a foraging device for pigs: once all the food was dispensed or the device contained no food, the pigs were not interested in using the device as it was primarily designed as a foraging device. A similar result was found by Vick *et al.* (2000) with zoo-housed macaque species. However, if the device had never dispensed food the pigs would have used it as a toy and the temporal patterning of its use would have been different – it would have been attractive as a toy and not as a source of food.

Thus, associating every type of environmental enrichment device with the delivery of food would be to deny the animals other forms of enrichment since they will react to all enrichment as if it were feeding or foraging enrichment. While for many species feeding and foraging behaviour occupy a large proportion of their time budget they are not the only behaviours expressed.

5.3.2 Use of non-food rewards

Food, as already stated, is a great motivator of animal behaviour but it is only one of a large number of potential reinforcers (i.e., rewards) that can be used. A powerful reinforcer of behaviour for many animals is social contact, e.g. stroking a dog for correct behaviour (Fogle, 1994; Pryor, 1985). It is important to realise that the world of captive animals is not and should not be governed by the application of food reinforcement. The reinforcing properties of stimuli differ, e.g. music (Lemercier, 2000; Gvaryahu *et al.*, 1989), toys (DeLeon *et al.*, 2000), nesting opportunity (Cooper & Appleby, 1997), social conspecific contact (Anderson, 1998), and other reinforcers such as those concerned with thermal comfort, comfort behaviour, the acquisition of water, should also be implemented. Thus, enrichment devices should be thought of in terms of the type of reinforcement with which an animal is provided. In a properly designed environmental enrichment programme (see Chapter 6) we seek to provide a wide range of types of reinforcement.

5.3.3 Implementing appropriate schedules of reward

The reinforcement schedule of animals can be thought of as when, where and how much behaviour is expressed in relation to the amount of reinforcement found. To take extremes, a lion may hunt successfully once every three days and acquire enough food to prevent hunger for several days. On the other hand, a sheep grazing on a field may be acquiring a constant amount of equally distributed food (in time and space). It is, therefore, important to understand these characteristics when designing an enrichment device. Inappropriate reinforcement schedules can result in animal-welfare problems. For example, the delivery of small amounts of food once every 30 seconds in a trough can cause schedule-induced behaviour, e.g. polydipsia (abnormal thirst). Pigs on such a schedule, while they are waiting for the next food reward, may pace up and down or perform other types of abnormal behaviour (Mason, 1991). Thus, reinforcement schedules are important in controlling the expression of a behaviour pattern. For example, variable reward schedules are highly effective at maintaining a high rate of expression of the rewarded behaviour (Chance, 1998).

5.4 Cosmetic Design Considerations

The importance of device cosmetics depends on the environment in which the device is to be used. In the case of laboratories and farms, device cosmetics are usually unimportant, here functionality in terms of animal welfare is of prime importance. The cosmetics of devices for pet animals mainly relate to human preferences for the device rather than animal preferences. In fact, we have no scientific evidence that animals possess aesthetic appreciation, however, we do know certain visual stimuli are more 'attractive' than others (see Chapter 10). The visual appearance of environmental enrichment devices can be important within the zoo environment. Research shows, overwhelmingly, that naturalistic type enclosures are much more effective at educating the public about the need for conservation. The reason is that naturalistic enclosures create an illusion of the animal living in the wild. Thus, the placing of an obviously made-man object within this environment shatters the illusion and reduces the educational value of the enclosure. Unfortunately, some zoos have thought that this means they can only use the naturalistic approach to environmental enrichment because the behavioural engineering approach usually uses man-made objects (see Chapter 1). Vick *et al.* (2000) demonstrated that it was possible to design an enrichment device, a puzzle feeder, that looked natural. The enrichment device was constructed from plastic fruit shapes (e.g. oranges, bananas, pears) that appeared natural within the enclosure.

5.4.1 Materials
The selection of materials to make an enrichment device is critical. Normally, the materials should have the following characteristics (Heidbrink, 1997):

- non toxic;
- thermally neutral, i.e. they do not take heat from the animal's body (compare holding stainless steel and plastic);
- tough, i.e. non shatterable when dropped, high tensile strength;
- water and cleaning-chemical proof;

- easily cleaned surface texture;
- able to withstand thermal stresses, i.e. will not crack or weaken when exposed to ambient or cleaning temperatures;
- able to be form strong joints with the same or other materials;
- non-glare finish.

5.4.2 Species considerations

It is important to recognise the differences between even closely related species when designing environmental enrichment devices, especially in relation to safety issues. A device that is safe in a capuchin enclosure will not necessarily be safe in a chimpanzee enclosure. For example, a hard plastic toy would facilitate play behaviour in both species but chimpanzees may throw it at other individuals, i.e. use it as a weapon. Thus, detailed knowledge of the particular species concerned is important when designing and implementing an enrichment device.

5.4.3 Enclosure considerations

The design of any environmental enrichment device must take into account the enclosure into which it is going to be implemented. This has serious consequences in terms of safety considerations (see below) and it may be possible to exploit certain features of the environment. In the example of the hunting enrichment device for cheetahs, Williams *et al.* (1996), took advantage of the enclosure's slope to design a hunting enrichment device that did not need a power source.

5.5 Safety Considerations

In the following two sections I have erred on the side of caution in the advice given, which I urge all people using newly-designed devices to do. I have found only three published cases of environmental enrichment devices causing safety problems. In case one, a plastic ball became lodged in the incisors of a rabbit (Shomer *et al.*, 2001). In the second case, the bedding material (cotton) caused conjunctivitis in nude mice (Bazille *et al.*, 2001). The third case involved a primate ingesting rope that was holding an enrichment device in place and this resulted in septic peritonitis (Hahn *et al.*, 2000). However, I know of several undocumented cases of enrichment devices or techniques causing injuries or harm to captive animals.

The following list of questions should be borne in mind when designing an environmental enrichment device and once the device is constructed this list should be consulted again. I cannot stress too highly the importance of animal safety. Remember, this list refers to the whole enrichment device, that includes locating ropes or chains, if used.

Has the device got any sharp edges?
Obviously, this would cause a safety risk. One simply needs to run a finger carefully along all surfaces and edges to assess this risk.

Can the animal's digits, limbs or other bodily appendages become trapped inside any part of the device?
Ideally, any holes in a device should be so small that the animal will not even attempt to insert a digit inside, or so large that a digit cannot become jammed in it. Obviously, one needs to know some basic animal physical statistics to ensure that there is no risk.

How likely is it that the animal could break the device?
It is important that the strength of an animal and its persistence in trying to break an enrichment device is never underestimated. I have been known to hit enrichment devices with a hammer to ensure they can withstand the abuse that chimpanzees and other powerful species can deliver.

If the device could be broken, would it break into sharp fragments or would the constituent parts of the device pose a safety risk?
It is obviously impossible to guarantee that an enrichment device will not be broken. Therefore, whenever possible, enrichment devices should be made of materials that do not shatter into sharp pieces.

Could the device be dismantled by the animal?
All the ape species have an amazing ability to undo nuts with their fingers or insert a fingernail into a screw head and turn the screw out. Therefore, the strength of all such connectors should be checked and where possible, nylon thread nuts should be used as they are nearly impossible to undo without a spanner.

If the device could be dismantled would any constituent parts pose a safety risk?
One should consider what could happen if the animal had access to the component parts of the enrichment device.

Can the device or any part of it be swallowed?
The size of the enrichment device is critical in terms of whether it could be swallowed; it is best to use as large a size as possible. If a device is made of cloth, could the animal extract long threads and consume them (this would cause gut impaction). When devices that are sewn together are used, a series of single stitches and not a running thread should be used.

Is the device made of non-toxic material?
As an obvious basic safety requirement, many materials in themselves, such as rope, may not be toxic but they may be soaked in an oil or other chemical that is

toxic. One should also consider whether the device needs to be covered in any lubricants and the toxicity of these.

Could the animal gnaw pieces off the device?
Rodents have teeth designed for gnawing and as such we need to consider whether they, or other species, could gnaw fragments from any device and ingest them.

Can the device be cleaned adequately or sterilised to prevent disease transmission?
It is important that an enrichment device does not become a haven or vector for pathogens, and so it should be made of waterproof, durable material that, ideally, has a smooth surface. If the device is to be sterilised using an autoclave, it must be able to withstand such treatment.

Can the animal in any way become entangled in the device?
There have been a number of primates that have become entangled in ropes in zoos and some individuals have been hanged. Experience in zoos shows that heavy gauge chain is less likely to become wrapped around an individual than rope. If ropes are used, then thicker ropes (e.g. ship ropes) are safer than thinner ropes. Finally, ropes should not be left dangling, both ends should be attached to a surface or structure.

Could the animal use the device as a weapon against cagemates, animal care-givers or other people, e.g. the public in a zoo?
A wide range of species with manipulative abilities have the potential to use environmental enrichment devices as a weapon. The animal may either strike another individual with the device or throw the device at another individual (the apes, some monkey species and elephants are all proficient throwers). Any device that could be used as a weapon should be secured to a point in the enclosure using a short chain. Ideally, the device should never have a pointed surface or shape. One should also consider the accidental use of an enrichment object as a weapon. (I have known male rhinos to accidentally toss a tractor tyre out of their enclosure, scattering the watching public.)

Could the animal use the device to damage its enclosure?
A number of species, especially apes, have learnt to take enrichment devices made of hard materials to the glass windows of their enclosures and hit at the corner of the window, sometimes breaking or shattering the window.

Could the animal use the device to facilitate escape from its enclosure?
The answer to this question often depends on the type of barriers being used to keep the animal inside its enclosure. Obvious things are long pieces of wood that can be used as ladders or ramps over physical barriers, e.g. moats and walls.

However, less obvious are plastic enrichment devices that can be used to negate the effects of electric fences or even be used to break electric fences.

Can the animal see the device?
Devices that move within an enclosure have the potential to cause an impact accident. For example, some zoos have experimented with putting heavy objects on a wire and pulley system for large ungulates, such as rhinos to knock flying along the wire. Obviously, the potential to strike an unwary bystander should be considered.

Are devices using electronics properly earthed and insulated?
A basic and obvious health requirement.

The safety assessment of an enrichment device does not stop once it has been safety tested (see below). Safety testing should be seen as a continuous process because of wear and tear on devices and because animals may discover unexpected ways of using a device. (Chimpanzees at Edinburgh Zoo had used plastic dustbin lids as toys on which to spin each other around, then after a few months one of them learnt to throw them frisbee-style at the public.)

Many institutions like to use recyclable materials as enrichment objects, most often as novel objects; examples include: clothing, shoes, books, magazines, cardboard tubes and cardboard boxes. It is best to remove all metal components from such objects, especially zips and staples. With clothing it is always worth considering the possibility that the animal can become trapped in it or put it on and not be able to take it off. On a more everyday level the following questions should always be considered.

Can the device be filled and maintained quickly?
Practical experience of working with environmental enrichment shows that only those devices that are quick to be filled and maintained will be implemented by animal care-givers, as often their time for enrichment activities is limited (see Chapter 6).

Does the installation of the device block any care-giver access or restrict view of the animals?
It is important that any enrichment device that is installed within an enclosure does not block the animal care-givers' exit or significantly reduce their ability to observe the animals.

Does use of the device require the care-giver to enter the enclosure?
The presence of an animal care-giver within the enclosure of some species can be a source of stress and therefore should be minimised. In the case of large dangerous species, the animal care-giver has only infrequent access to the animal enclo-

sure and, therefore, an enrichment device that needs filling, cleaning, etc. every day would be a problem. This problem could be solved by training the animal to go inside in response to a whistle or verbal command.

Is the device of the simplest design possible?
The simpler the design of the device, e.g. the fewer moving parts and electronics it has, the less likely that it will breakdown and need repairing. In addition, when simple devices become broken it is usually possible to repair them without the use of a specialist.

5.5.1 Product testing

Once you have followed the safety checklist above, then comes the time to product-test the finished device before it is given to the animals. The product testing should be done by the animal care-givers that work with the animals concerned and the institution's veterinarian. Product testing for animals should follow the same product-testing procedures that are used for the toys of young children. (In fact, the enrichment-device tester at Los Angeles Zoo, USA, actually works for a major children's toy manufacturing company.) The basic tests to perform on the finished product are:

- drop test (the device is dropped from one metre high onto a concrete floor);
- sharp seams and edge test;
- the strength of attachments, i.e. can they be pulled off;
- the strength of seams.

The first time a device is placed within an enclosure it must be done within a situation that the animal care-giver can control in case the device has to be quickly removed. In the case of dangerous animals, it is useful to have a way of moving them out of the enclosure where the enrichment device is being introduced, e.g. be in possession of food treats that can be used to lure the animal to another area or alternative enclosure. The animal care-giver needs to have the time to spend watching the animal use the device and normally, after a few hours of being in the enclosure, the device should be removed. Removal of the device occurs for two reasons: (1) safety of the animal (we need time and repeated exposures to establish the device's safety); (2) to check the condition of the device. Even if you are using a commercially produced environmental enrichment device I would strongly recommend using the safety procedures outlined in this chapter before implementing it.

5.6 Discussion and Summary of the Product Design Process

The design of environmental enrichment devices is a complex and often long duration process. It is important to question whether the time, energy and money put into device design is cost-effective. If the same effects could be achieved by a change in husbandry method then the answer would be no. The design of an enrichment device should, therefore, only take place when there is no other husbandry or management method to solicit the desired behaviour patterns (see the pig and cheetah examples above).

The product design process can be summarised as:

(1) Define purpose;
>> What is the purpose of the item being designed?
>> Why design it?
(2) Define design parameters and constraints;
>> Stresses, size, weight, cost, safety factor, materials, cosmetics, etc.
(3) Research and analyse similar items:
>> What are their good and bad points?
(4) Prioritise design parameters and constraints in order of importance:
>> (i)   cost,
>> (ii)   safety,
>> (iii) weight,
>> (iv)   cosmetics.
(5) Create a preliminary sketch of the overall design:
>> Helps focus independent parts to achieve goal.
(6) Quick structural analysis of design:
>> Look at potential areas of weakness, such as attachments, seams and areas that will receive physical stress, e.g. fulcrums and load bearing parts.
(7) If possible, create solid models of individual parts and assemblies.
(8) Check for functional problems.
(9) Check the feasibility of constructing the device.
(10) Run preliminary safety checks:
>> (i)   verify that the device conforms to safety limits.
>> (ii)   If there is a problem, redesign and reanalyse parts.
(11) Create final device drawings.
(12) Assemble parts for prototype device.
(13) Physically test parts to determine failure points:
>> (i)   if failure stress exceeds safety factor limits, then the design is good.
>> (ii) if part fails below safety limit, go to step 6.
(14) Test the device with animal under controlled conditions:
>> (i)   if device fails go to step 6.
(15) Write the final design down with full details.

The Enrichment Programme 6

In this chapter I will discuss the implementation and management of an environmental enrichment programme. On one level we might wish an enrichment programme only to verify that we are providing the best conditions possible for animals in our care. In certain institutions an enrichment programme helps to motivate staff and provides evidence to external scrutiny that the institution has an active programme. In the US, enrichment programmes are a legal requirement for institutions that house primates (see Chapter 1).

6.1 Setting Goals

An effective enrichment programme must have a set of goals or objectives. In a zoo environment these goals might be: (1) the maintenance of behavioural competence; or (2) full expression of natural behaviour patterns. Whereas, for a household pet, the goal might simply be to provide an environment in which the animal will experience the optimum level of welfare. The aforementioned goals are obviously very general but when working with individual animals we should have specific goals, e.g. to provide farmed mink with the opportunity to express hunting behaviour. The importance of a goal is that it sets out what we are trying to achieve and creates a focus for our activities. Once we have our general and specific goals we can start the process of choosing (see Chapters 8–11) and designing environmental enrichment (see Chapter 5) for our target animals. It is important to remember that in a social group certain types of enrichment may only be effective for some group members, tool-using enrichment for chimpanzees (only good for females), for example. Thus, the targets of enrichment must be thought about within a social group, as must the provision of sufficient enrichment for animals to have access to it. Insufficient access to enrichment, at best, might cause frustration in those individuals denied access and, at worst, it might cause fighting (see Chapter 5).

If we are introducing new enrichment to an existing enclosure we need to think carefully about how we are going to do this. In the past, many enrichment devices were placed in an area that the animal utilised the most. Presumably, the animal care-giver hoped that this would increase the use of the enrichment. (I think this choice of location tends to reflect the desire of the care-giver to see the results of their work, rather than what is best for the animal.) For species that are naturally neophobic, e.g. most bird species, or those that have been reared in unchanging environments, the introduction of an enrichment device can be stressful. The animals' initial reaction to the enrichment device may be one of fear, we might see the animals move as far away from the device as possible (Timmermans *et al.*, 1994; Mitchell *et al.*, 1981). They may not approach or interact with the enrichment device for several days. It is therefore vital when we introduce an environmental enrichment device that it is placed in a relatively unimportant part of the enclosure as far as the animal is concerned. Certainly not the centre of the enclosure, nor near any resources such as food or water, and not near sleeping or resting sites.

In my experience working within zoos, I have often found zoo keepers to be impatient to see animals using an enrichment device. I have found it wise, therefore, to explain to animal care-givers that they should give the animals time and definitely not remove the enrichment after only a few hours or days. I remember one example where a keeper wished to remove a foraging enrichment device from a tapir's enclosure because the animal had not used it all day. After a long discussion I persuaded the keeper to leave the device within the enclosure overnight as I knew tapirs forage principally at night; the next morning the foraging device was empty of food. Once the keeper saw that his efforts had not been in vain he was very happy, albeit disappointed not to see the tapir actually using the enrichment device. It is definitely a harder decision to leave enrichment in an animal's enclosure if it is obviously causing fear, especially if the animal is housed in a very small enclosure. However, we need to think about the long-term benefits that the animal should accrue from the enrichment (repeated exposure to novelty reduces an animal's general level of fear; see Chapters 3 and 11).

The key component of any environmental enrichment programme is the people who work with, and are responsible for the well-being of the animals. For an enrichment programme to be successful, the people working within it need to be motivated, educated and empowered. People can be motivated in a variety of ways. The Night Safari in Singapore motivates its staff with financial incentives to produce stimulating environments. Evidence of good enrichment work with animals could form part an animal care-giver's staff appraisal and be linked to promotion. Other institutions provide motivators, such as sending their best staff to environmental enrichment conferences. I believe that all institutions that utilise animals must have a scheme to motivate their workers to implement environmental enrichment. It is vital that in the case of any positive publicity about enrichment, the people who did the work receive the credit. Perhaps the biggest disincentive for anyone is having someone else take, or be given credit for their work; this often requires careful handling of journalists. (I have learnt over the years that you must insist with journalists to see a copy of what they are going to publish before it is published.)

It is important that all animal care-givers receive basic education about animal welfare (see Chapter 13 for a list of resources such as courses), this can be done formally or informally. The next step is to set up an enrichment group, circle or committee (although I prefer not to use the word committee as for many people it has negative connotations), which should have an open membership, within an institution. The group should be set the task of achieving the institution's goals in relation to environmental enrichment. To this end, the group should meet regularly to discuss what needs to be done to achieve the institution's enrichment goals; I have found this is best done by having an open discussion session at each meeting. Meetings can also be convened for invited outside experts to talk about their work, experience or research with environmental enrichment. Such groups obviously need access to information about enrichment (see Chapter 13) and this usually means they will need a budget to buy books, magazines, videos etc. On the subject of money, while environmental enrichment can be inexpensive, it is usually not free and a budget is needed for this vital activity. Finally, the activities and achievements of this group should be communicated within an institution and to the outside world, i.e. to the media.

Too much bureaucracy can stop an environmental enrichment programme dead. I remember going to a famous large zoo and being disappointed to see little environmental enrichment. I managed to find a zoo keeper to talk to and eventually got on to the subject of environmental enrichment. I asked the keeper if he knew about the subject, which he did in great detail. Then unprompted, he apologised for the lack of enrichment but explained to me that it took him six months to get permission to give a plastic ball to a marine mammal species. He explained that every enrichment device had to be approved by various committees, he listed six to me! My experience is that bureaucracy such as this is a strong de-motivator but nor is it wise to allow anyone to implement environmental enrichment without discussing it with other people. Animals have been injured by environmental enrichment devices in the past (see Chapter 5 for examples). The aforementioned enrichment group would be the ideal forum to discuss new forms of enrichment as the group should consist of animal care-givers, their managers and veterinary surgeons, thereby, providing a good evaluation of the enrichment idea in a short-time period. The safety considerations for environmental enrichment are discussed in Chapter 5 which gives a checklist of questions to ask.

6.2 The Enrichment Diary

Enrichment that is added to an enclosure rather than being an integral part of the enclosure should be recorded in an enrichment diary. The enrichment diary provides a record of what enrichment the animal has received (the enrichment should be described in the institution's enrichment manual see below), the diary also functions to ensure that the animals receive a variety of enrichment that is varied over time. I recommend that the following information should be recorded:

- Date,
- Species,
- Enclosure,
- Environmental enrichment (name of enrichments used),
- Assessment of enrichment use (subjective assessment of the animals' use of the environmental enrichment on a scale of 1 to 10),
- Comments (anything unusual or special that happened),
- Name and signature (I believe that signing a diary page encourages people to take it more seriously).

If the institution has the money, this information should be recorded on a computer diary programme, such as a database or spreadsheet programme, as this would facilitate analysis of the enrichment programme (for examples see the Disney web site listed in Chapter 13). All enrichment programmes should be analysed for their effectiveness. In the ideal world this would consist of making systematic behavioural studies on each enrichment with each species, clearly completely impractical. However, the subjective assessments of enrichment of how much animals use enrichment by animal care-givers can provide us with information about the relative effectiveness of enrichment over time. Such diaries could be expanded to include behavioural assessments (Mellen, 1994), for example, on a subjective scale of 1 to 10 of how often the animal performs abnormal behaviour. In a zoo environment, the diary could record the general impression of visitors to the enrichment, e.g. unaware, negative, neutral and positive. Of course, I recognise that for institutions housing huge numbers of the same species, farms, for example, the recording of individual data would be impossible. However, a small sample of animals in different enclosures could be observed.

6.3   The Enrichment Manual

In conjunction with an enrichment diary I think it would be useful for each institution to have an environmental enrichment manual, a book that describes all the types of enrichment employed by the institution. This book should have the possibility to be expanded as new ideas are implemented, so a binder format might be most appropriate. The following format was devised by Gordon McLeod at Edinburgh Zoo, and subsequently copied by Marwell Zoo, UK, (see Chapter 13) through conversations with zoo keepers.

Category	Description
Method or Device	Title of the enrichment technique.
Design and Implementation	A brief description of the actual device or technique (e.g. size, position within enclosure) and how it is implemented.
Species	The individual species or groups (e.g. felids, ungulates) with which the method has been used. The evaluations of the method are based on the response of the animals mentioned in this category.
Purpose	The reasons for implementing the device or technique, e.g. to provide exercise, sensory stimulation or to encourage natural behaviour.
Advantages	Main good points about the technique, including its practicality or aspects of the species husbandry that make the method particularly appropriate.
Disadvantages	Main negative points about the technique, including possible risks, husbandry problems and general drawbacks.
Improvements	Possible ways in which the technique may work more effectively or other methods that can be used in conjunction, e.g. alternative designs or varying location.
Comments	Other additional information that may be useful, based upon practical experience of the method.
Frequency of Use	How often the method is employed, e.g. constantly (for permanent features), daily, once a week, or for set periods of time.
Ratings	Methods are rated from 1 to 10 (10 = Best) in four categories. If the method is used for many different species in one zoo section, e.g. primates, an average rating should be used. Where several sections use the same method, separate ratings should be provided for each section.
Usefulness	How well the technique achieves its goals.
Convenience	How easy the technique is to implement from the perspective of being time consuming or awkward for care-givers to use.

Value for Money	How much the technique or device cost to make or maintain, whether the device is considered a good investment and a success with the animals.
Range of Users	Relative proportion (scale 1 to 10) of animals using the enrichment technique. A single animal in a group would score 1; if most animals used the technique it would score 6–7. If all animals of all species listed use the enrichment, it would score 10.
Contributors	The names of the people and their section within the institution that contributed the information.

Below is a typical example of a completed enrichment manual page.

Method or Device	Kebab feeder.
Design and Implementation	Fruits, vegetables or nuts are threaded onto a length of thick metal wire. One end is hooked onto the roof of the enclosure (or the wire is bent into a circle), around a rope or onto a branch. In the case of nuts, a nail and hammer are used to create holes in individual nuts through which the wire can pass.
Species	Parrot species and frugivorous bats.
Purpose	Novel method of food presentation that requires birds and bats to free fruit, vegetables or nuts from a mobile object. It makes feeding more challenging and physically demanding.
Advantages	Position can be varied within enclosure, determining accessibility and therefore ease of use. Maintains the interest of bats and birds for a considerable length of time. Very easy to construct device that requires no maintenance.
Disadvantages	Fruit and vegetables once cut or, in the case of nuts, once the shell has been cracked, will rot relatively quickly. Difficult to assemble nuts onto device. Dropped fruit, vegetables and shell fragments can create mess.

Improvements
Comments   If the kebab feeder is located so that it cannot be
                                 accessed via moving along branches, the bats or
                                 birds are required to fly to the device. The nuts are
                                 subsequently removed whilst hanging from the mesh
                                 ceiling, making the device much more taxing.

Frequency of Use   A least once per week for both parrots and bats.

Ratings out of 10 for:
Usefulness   8   **Convenience**   7
Value for Money   10   **Range of users**   10

Contributed by   Jo Bloggs, the Bird Section.

The enrichment manual should be widely available within the institution, and
should be used in conjunction with the enrichment diary to ensure that animals
are receiving a variety of types of environmental enrichment. It is very tempting
just to provide animals with four or five types of enrichment that we know work
well but repeated, frequent presentation may devalue a particular type of enrichment (see section on toys in Chapter 11). The enrichment manual is also an
excellent medium for sharing and exchanging ideas with other institutions. It also
provides evidence of the seriousness of the institution about environmental enrichment, something that should be important to any institution.

6.4 Changing Animal Care-giver Attitudes

The final subject I wish to include is about changing animal care-givers' attitudes.
In my experience, most animal care-givers work with animals because they find
the job highly rewarding (and not for the salary!). Some people make this type of
work a lifelong career. I have often encountered animal care-givers with more than
20 years of experience. In institutions that are commencing environmental enrichment programmes, these people need to be educated in a careful manner about the
need for environmental enrichment. It might be true that the way the institution
has kept the animals for the last 20 years or more is not good for animal welfare
but this information needs to be phrased very carefully. If you present this information as only factual scientific information, then in my experience, you will upset
and alienate some animal care-givers. Basically, they will perceive this new information as a criticism of their animal care. Remember, they entered the job to look
after animals, so such perceived criticism can be like saying you have done your
job badly for the last 20 years. It is much better to present such information by
discussing how animals are currently managed. What do they think about this or
that (the positive and negative aspects)? What would they like to change? What

improvements do they think are necessary? What support would they need to make such changes? The new information should be presented in this format because it recognises the skills of the animal care-givers and values their experience. Unfortunately, some people who have tried to effect changes in institutions simply have not had the interpersonal skills to do so. I have seen many cases where a consultant on animal welfare has come into an institution and basically pointed the finger of blame at people for managing animals in less than optimal animal welfare friendly environments. The result of this is usually that the staff will do everything in their power not to implement new ideas, such as environmental enrichment. Thus, education needs to be seen not only as a system of conveying information but also as a means of changing and modifying attitudes. Once we have modified and educated existing staff, the next step is to consider the environment within which new staff will be working. Take the role of the zoo keeper, historically the job of the zoo keeper was to feed the animals and to keep their enclosures clean. (As a historical note, many zoos, up to the 1970s, had enclosure inspections one day per week – this interesting piece of sociology perhaps reflects the large number of ex-army officers that became zoo directors after World War II. In the UK, Edinburgh Zoo even had daily uniform inspections!) A new zoo keeper needs to be taught that recent activities, such as environmental enrichment, are as integral to the job as feeding and cleaning the animal. Such activities must never be presented as additional work; to prevent this, some zoos use the term 'environmental husbandry' instead of enrichment to relate this activity to the well established term animal husbandry.

6.5 Conclusion

I always remember a zoo keeper at the 3rd International Conference on Environmental Enrichment who said: 'The following people in the zoo can stop enrichment from happening; the director, the curator and, most importantly, the zoo keeper'. Thus, elegantly illustrating that everyone in an institution must be motivated, educated and empowered to implement environmental enrichment. Environmental enrichment is the responsibility of everyone who works within an institution that utilises animals and I would argue that the public also have a responsibility to ensure its implementation since they are the ultimate consumers of the institutions' products.

Enrichment for Different Categories of Animals

Each of the four main categories of captive animals, namely, companion (pets), farm, laboratory and zoo, has its own special requirements and restrictions when it comes to the application of environmental enrichment. In this chapter I will discuss these special requirements and restrictions.

7.1 Companion Animals

The range of animals we now keep as pets in our houses is quite broad and is continuing to expand. The species commonly kept include: birds, cats, dogs, fish, reptiles, rodents and insects (I am not covering insects in this book). I will cover horses in the section on farm animals because they are not kept within our houses. Unfortunately, we have virtually no information on the welfare of these species within the home environment. People normally only become concerned about the welfare of their pet when it is physically injuring itself, for example, fur and feather plucking in mammals and birds, respectively. The reason why we do not investigate the psychological well-being of companion animals is something that is not understood. It has been suggested to me by various scientists that the topic is too controversial and emotionally charged to touch because we are often talking about a 'loved family member'. Thus, to imply the welfare of a pet animal is not good would be perceived by the owner as a direct criticism. There seems to be an unspoken sentiment that because we 'love' our companion animals then their welfare must be good. Yet, in the UK and North America the number of consultants dealing with behavioural problems is growing at a rapid rate; there are books on the subject in most languages and television programmes that specifically deal with such problems (Appleby, 1998; Bohnenkamp, 1994; Campbell, 1995; Dodman, 1997; Neville, 1993; Wright & Lashnits, 1994).

Table 7.1 Abnormal behaviours expressed by companion animals.

Species	Abnormal Behaviour
Birds	Repetitive pecking at the same spot, somersaulting on the perch, head bobbing, repetitive route tracing.
Rodents	Somersaulting, repetitive route tracing.
Dogs	Wall bouncing, repetitive barking, repetitive route tracing.
Cats	Repetitive route tracing.
Reptiles	Glass rubbing.

All this suggests that the level of welfare problems for companion animals is not insignificant. Although the majority of the public perhaps, see such behavioural problems as a failure of the animal and not of the way that they house and manage the animal. In the world of horse owners, behavioural problems such as crib biting or wind sucking are described as behavioural vices, a clear attempt to put the blame on the animal and not on the owner (Winskill *et al.*, 1995; Winskill *et al.*, 1996). The abilities of the public in western societies to recognise abnormal behaviour in zoo animals is quite good, if the comments in zoo visitor books are anything to go by. However, the same people often fail to recognise physically similar behaviours in their pets (Table 7.1), but it seems that 'love' makes them blind (Zasloff & Hart, 1998; Archer, 1997). Clearly, despite what pet owners think 'love' is not enough to ensure that a pet experiences a good level of animal welfare.

Most species that we keep as pets are also used in one or more of the other categories of animal keeping. Domestic dogs are used extensively in toxicology studies in laboratories across the world and several types of rodent species are used as laboratory animals (Poole, 1999). The domestic rabbit can be a farm species and a laboratory species as well as a companion animal. Exotic species of birds and species of reptiles may also be housed in the zoo environment. Thus, although we may have no information on the species' welfare in the home, we often have information about its captive housing requirements and sometimes excellent systematic welfare studies. The welfare of domestic dogs in laboratories has been widely studied, and most studies conclude that the two most enriching things we can provide are a human to play with and exercise the dog, and other dogs for companionship (Loveridge, 1998; Hubrecht, 1993; Rooney *et al.*, 2000; Rooney & Bradshaw, 2002). Despite this, we live in societies where pet dogs are often left alone for prolonged periods of the day which results in behaviour problems such as separation anxiety (Seksel & Lindeman, 2001; Flannigan & Dodman, 2001; Simpson, 2000; Lund & Jorgensen, 1999; Appleby, 1993; Voith & Borchelt, 1985; Takeuchi *et al.*, 2000). Behavioural information for a particular species may have more relevance for pet animals rather than zoo or laboratory animals. For example, one of the biggest problems in dog shelters and laboratory dog houses is barking, but this is caused by housing large numbers of dogs within auditory, olfactory and visual contact of one another, a situation that does not occur to the same extent within the companion animal environment (Wells & Hepper, 2000a; Lund & Jorgensen, 1999; Wells & Hepper, 2000b). The laboratories of companies producing food for companion animals may provide the best data on the welfare of this category of animal since they usually strive to house their animals in home-like conditions (Loveridge, 1998; McCune, 1997).

Most companion animals receive two types of environmental enrichment, human–animal contact (i.e. social enrichment) and toys (i.e. object enrichment) (Podberscek, 1997; Serpell, 1996; Jagoe & Serpell, 1996; Rooney et al., 2000; Hubrecht, 1993; Evans, 2001; Steinigeweg, 2000). In Chapter 9 I discuss the value of human–animal contact as a substitute for housing animals in social groups. In the case of pets, human–animal contact may unwittingly be of a stressful nature. Firstly, the human may not have a good understanding of how to touch, stroke or pick up an animal, this is usually the case with young children who should always be supervised in such activities (Fogle, 1994). Secondly, for some species human handling is completely inappropriate because the species perceives the human as a predator, small lizards, for example (Kreger & Mench, 1993). Many humans believe that if an animal is not enjoying being petted then it would struggle and attempt to escape from them. However, many species when captured by a predator 'freeze' to feign death, or freeze when a predator is close. Unfortunately, the calm behaviour of such animals in human hands makes the owner believe the experience is enriching to the animal. In the Antarctic, nesting penguins show no behavioural response to the approach of humans, however, if we measure their heart rate we find it triples as humans approach (Culik & Wilson, 1995; Nimon et al., 1996). We cannot take non-avoidance of human contact as meaning that the species 'enjoys' human–animal interactions. As a final comment on this subject, species that use cryptic camouflage to avoid predation usually avoid predators by freezing, which is associated with high levels of stress (Korte, 2001). Thus, if we are handling such a species we need to be sure that this is a positive experience for the animal. I do, however, strongly believe that human–animal interaction for some species, especially solitary kept dogs, is the main source of psychological buffering the animal receives if they have been properly socialised (see Chapter 9).

The pet market is awash with toys for almost every species that is kept. Unfortunately, human adults usually buy the toys, therefore, most pet toys are marketed to be attractive to human adults rather than to the pet. Let me illustrate with the example of children's teddy bears; the teddy bear has evolved to a particular shape and form (big head, flat face and short fat limbs) because human adults find these characteristics attractive (Sternglanz et al., 1977). Studies on children of less than eight years of age show that they are not concerned with the physical characteristics of the teddy bear (Morris et al., 1995). It would be interesting to see how much work a companion animal would be prepared to do to get access to different types of toys using the methodologies I outlined in Chapter 4. A study on farmed mink showed that they were not prepared to work hard to have access to toys (Cooper & Mason, 2000). Toys, as discussed in Chapter 11, have only a limited ability to enrich an animal's life. In the case of pets, I think money could be more wisely spent on other types of environmental enrichment (see Chapters 8 to 11).

The pet owner needs to think more about the psychological well-being of their animal. To make improvements in their pet's welfare, owners obviously need much more information. There exist many books about the captive maintenance of nearly every species that is kept as a pet animal (see Chapter 13). The quality of these books varies enormously, one strategy to select the best book is to see if there is a society for the keeping of a given species in captivity and ask them which book they recommend. In addition, I would recommend reading books about the species' natural history; for some species this will be the natural history of their closest genetic relative, e.g. the wolf in the case of domestic dogs.

7.2 Farm Animals

On a personal note, I find environmental enrichment and animal welfare for farm animal species perhaps the most frustrating area of animal welfare. Most of the best experimental studies into animal welfare have been conducted on farm animal species; the theoretical understanding of animal welfare has been advanced massively by scientists that principally work with farm animal species (Appleby & Hughes, 1997). Without doubt our knowledge about the welfare of farm animals is the most advanced of any category of animal. Yet, the application of this knowledge with farm animals is minimal. Mench (1998) has noted that farm animals live in extremely barren enclosures; even the best of such environments appear barren in comparison with the average unenriched zoo enclosures.

There are a number of reasons why there is so much research on farm animal welfare and so little implementation. The number one factor is undoubtedly economics (Webster, 2001; McGlone, 2001; van Veen, 1999; Asheim & Eik, 1998; Waterhouse, 1996; Webster, 1982; McInerney, 1991). The number of animals used to produce food is enormous; for example, the UK (population c. 58 million) normally has around 40 million laying hens to produce its eggs, in excess of 100 million broilers to produce its chicken, and in excess of 20 million fattening pigs to produce pork and bacon. Animal food producers typically work on small profit margins, therefore, they are extremely sensitive to things that affect the cost of their product. For example, the profit on a single broiler hen can be as low as a few pence and through market fluctuations, farmers can lose money on each animal. The other consequence of low profit margins is that due to economies of scale, most animals are produced in huge intensive units that often house thousands of animals. In most Western countries the image of the farmer with his dozen cows, a handful of chickens and twenty pigs is no longer a reality. Thus, any form of environmental enrichment, if it is to be adopted, must not affect the profitability of animal production. The main ways that profitability can be affected are: the cost of buying an enrichment device, increased labour costs due to the enrichment device, and increased costs due to hygiene or other related management practices associated with the enrichment device.

One potential solution to the economic restrictions on environmental enrichment is to increase the cost of the product and thereby generate money that can be used to house animals in more enriched environments. This is the approach that the UK based charity the RSPCA has taken with its welfare-friendly marketing of its 'Freedom Foods' animal products (Kells *et al.*, 2001). The market for such premium-priced food products, even in an animal-welfare conscious country like the UK, has proven to be small. Most of the public are not, it seems, prepared financially to support the animal welfare-friendly strategies that they verbally support (Bennett, 1996, 1997, 1998). Part of the reason is obviously financial – not everyone in society can afford to buy premium priced products. The other part of the reason is that most people live in urban societies with no contact with animals and, to a large extent, are ignorant of how they are produced (Serpell, 1999; Bellaver & Bellaver, 1999). Perhaps one solution would be to develop a public education programme to help consumers make an informed choice; however, such a programme is unlikely to be popular with most animal producers.

Governments cannot legislate to force its people to buy welfare-friendly products at a premium price. The UK, for example, banned the production of tethered pigs in stalls but it cannot ban the importation of pig meat produced in this system. The World Trade Organization (WTO) does not permit one country to force its standards of product production on another country (Gregory, 2000; Korthals, 2001; Brooman & Legge, 2000). The most famous example is the production of dolphin 'unfriendly' tuna in Mexico: the WTO did not allow the US to ban the importation of this product. Ultimately, cheap food policies have proved to be extremely popular around the world and for this reason alone, governments are unlikely to support initiatives that will increase product price (McInerney, 1991; DenOuden *et al.*, 1997; Hartung, 2000). So there seems to be no simple, political solution to the problem.

I believe that many farm animal-welfare scientists are also different from zoo or laboratory animal-welfare scientists in their unconscious motivation to see the application of welfare-friendly systems. These scientists have experimental units and a few experimental farms that they visit to conduct their experiments. Zoo and laboratory animal-welfare scientists have their offices surrounded by animals and spend their working life seeing the animals in their captive environments. Perhaps, therefore, they have a greater level of motivation to effect animal-welfare changes. Farmers, of course, work with their animals everyday and it is undisputed that most of them care about their animals. However, given the inevitable death of their animals, farmers try and avoid thinking about the plight of their animals by using so called distancing devices, such as not naming animals. Many farmers report feeling that they are not in control of the animal production process, which they view as very hierarchical (Serpell, 1999).

Enrichment for farm animals has tended therefore, to focus on the design of better environments such as modified cages for hens (Barnett & Newman, 1997; Lindberg & Nicol, 1997; Appleby, 1997) and family-pen systems for pigs (Smidt *et al.*, 1992; Stolba & Wood-Gush, 1984; Arey, 1997). It should be noted that even these systems are unenriched in comparison with the average unenriched zoo enclosure (Mench, 1998). Few of these welfare-friendly systems have been commercially adopted because most of them produce a more expensive, and arguably, therefore, a premium-priced product. If the premium-priced product was of better quality, one could perhaps find a bigger market for it but the improvements in quality due to welfare-friendly housing systems are minimal (see Chapter 3). Of course, there are still a few small-scale, family-run animal-production businesses where the farmer can implement environmental enrichment. (I have seen many pig farms in Sweden where the farmer has developed his own housing system to improve the welfare of his animals but, unfortunately, the Swedes are the exception and not the rule). Principally, this type of farming exists in less-developed countries and as economies in such countries improve welfare-friendly systems are likely to vanish, as in the West (Bellaver & Bellaver, 1999).

The picture I paint of farm animal welfare and environmental enrichment is unfortunately black but perhaps by illuminating the problems we can attempt to find solutions. The knowledge of how to enrich farm animals' lives exists, we just need to find a way to implement it. I should perhaps finish by saying that advances are being made and potentially more welfare-friendly systems are being adopted. The UK saw a large increase in outdoor pig production in the 1990s but extensive systems are not the panacea they appear to be (Matthews, 1996; Hemsworth *et al.*, 1995; Oldigs *et al.*, 1995a; Oldigs *et al.*, 1995b; Horrell *et al.*, 2001). Often, the change to such systems just changes the nature of the welfare problems, e.g. restriction of physical movement in the case of indoor pigs, or outdoor pigs who suffer from exposure to the weather. Outdoor pigs have more freedom to express more normal patterns of behaviour but their freedom from thermal discomfort has been compromised. In fact, many outdoor pigs are nose-ringed to prevent rooting, therefore, their increase in natural behaviour is not as great as it should be (Horrell *et al.*, 2001). Clearly, the situation for improving farm-animal welfare is difficult but this should not dissuade us from attempting to implement changes that can improve animal welfare, such as environmental enrichment.

7.3 Laboratory Animals

Globally, tens of millions of animals are housed each year within a laboratory environment. Nearly, 90% of these animals are rats or mice, the rest being composed of a mixture of animals that also includes dogs and primates. The vast majority of these animals are used in toxicology studies. Most countries in the world have laws requiring that all products that are consumed by humans or animals (e.g. medicines or food) or come into physical contact with humans or animals (e.g. household cleaning products, such as oven cleaner) have their constituent chemical components' toxicologically tested (Knierim & Jackson, 1997; Brooman & Legge, 1997). The rest of the animals are used for biomedical research (e.g. drug development) and fundamental research (e.g. studies into how the nervous system works).

The most important factor in all laboratory animal research is the production of accurate results. To this end most laboratory animals are housed within highly climate-controlled environments. In the case of medical research, these environments can also be highly sterile. The species used has often been bred to produce individuals that are highly genetically similar (an inbred line) to reduce interindividual variation. The housing is typically identical for all animals in the same experiment. Many governments prescribe by law the minimum housing requirements for laboratory animals. In the UK, the Home Office publishes these requirements and through its inspectorate service ensures that they are adhered to (see *http://www.homeoffice.gov.uk*). These are the kind of constraints that we often encounter within a laboratory animal house.

Unless the experimental protocols are extremely strict, is usually possible within the laboratory house to implement a lot of environmental enrichment. In the UK, the Home Office inspectors actively encourage laboratories to use as much environmental enrichment as possible. Much of the laboratory-animal community has long realised that testing the toxicology of a chemical on a highly stressed animal is not as accurate as testing on an unstressed animal (Poole, 1997). Thus, although environmental enrichment can create more varied environments, it can help to produce much more accurate results (see Chapter 2).

The profit margins involved in the development of new drugs by pharmaceutical companies can be enormous. Therefore, laboratories face less financial restrictions than farms. However, one unfortunate characteristic they do share with farms in the economy of scale is the use of small rodents. A laboratory might typically house 50 to 200 dogs and 10 000 to 50 000 mice (usually housed in cages of five individuals). It is physically difficult for any laboratory to provide daily enrichment for each mouse cage. Mouse cages also tend to be small due to the cost of producing and maintaining controlled-environment rooms. Thus, in terms of enrichment for small laboratory rodents, we need to be concentrating on features built into their cage, or developing novel welfare friendly environments. Dogs and primates tend to be afforded much more space. Perhaps because people are much more concerned about their psychological well-being in comparison to that of a mouse (Ings *et al.*, 1997; Ryder, 1989; Zasloff, 1996).

I have been privileged to visit many laboratory-animal houses in the UK and have been universally impressed by the standards of animal welfare that I have observed. The primate houses of some laboratories are as good as most zoo primate enclosures. The one sad piece of information I need to relay is that some of these laboratory animal houses could be even better if it were not for animal-rights activists (see Chapter 1). In the UK, animal-rights activists through their, in my opinion, misguided activities have denied all species of laboratory animal the opportunity to have outdoor enclosures, which in the case of dogs and primates would be very beneficial (Brent *et al.*, 1991; Keeling & Duncan, 1991; O'Neill *et al.*, 1991). Fortunately, the oppressive activities of animal rights activists on animal housing are restricted to just a few countries (Spira, 1991; Regan, 1984; Bekoff, 1997). Ironically, these activists often are strongest in the countries with the best animal welfare laws, such as the UK. It is to be hoped that such activists do not force all laboratory-animal experiments to be conducted in countries with lower animal-welfare standards. It is also sad that the activists have, to an extent, made laboratory animal-house workers more remote from the rest of the animal-welfare community (the details of their conferences in the UK are secret, for example). I know that they have a lot to contribute and would benefit from an interchange of ideas with other animal workers.

7.4 Zoo Animals

Zoos are not only unique in the number of different species they house but also in terms of their exposure to public scrutiny. I can think of no other animal institutions that actively display their animals to the public. A consequence of this public attention is the pressure that the public can exert when it wants changes. It is well known that since the 1970s zoos have evolved from mere collections of animals to captive breeding (conservation orientated) centres. In this same period of time they have become serious about protecting the welfare of the animals they care for (Bostock, 1993; Tudge, 1992). Personally, I think it is irrelevant whether zoos have adopted or been forced to adopt new goals so long as they are genuinely trying to achieve these goals.

Zoos have the greatest opportunities to implement environmental enrichment of all four categories of animals discussed in this chapter. The only major constraint some zoos face is the lack of money. However, given that they are working with relatively small numbers of animals, even financially poor zoos can afford to implement environmental enrichment. I have seen some very poor zoos, in terms of animal welfare, in rich Western countries and some excellent zoos in developing countries. In my experience of running training courses in environmental enrichment around the world, it is not the wealth of the country that determines whether environmental enrichment is implemented but the will and drive of the zoo professionals to do so. It is not surprising, therefore, that the greatest sources of ideas about environmental enrichment come from zoos (see Chapters 8–11 and 13). The type of enrichment a zoo implements can, however, be restricted by the goals of the zoo itself. Modern zoos typically have four goals: conservation, education, research and recreation (Bostock, 1993; Tudge, 1992). The poorer zoos in the world are often not so constrained by such goals and can put functional environmental enrichment as their priority, whereas the implementation of naturalistic environmental enrichment is much more expensive. It is ultimately better that animals receive enrichment, even if this means the ability to educate the public is reduced through the enrichment being of an inappropriate type (Catlow, 1997).

A zoo that is heavily focussed on using its animals in environmental education programmes is most likely to house its animals in naturalistic exhibits and will not wish to use anthropogenic objects or materials within the animal's enclosures (Kreger *et al.*, 1998). Even if providing chimpanzees with cardboard boxes to destroy was the best enrichment in the world for this species, it would probably not be permitted in a zoo with environmental education as its primary goal. In fact, in the US the AZA strongly recommends only naturalistic enrichment for naturalistic enclosures. Alternatively, a zoo that is heavily focussed on field conservation and re-introduction would put great emphasis on environments that maintain their animals' behavioural competence. Thus, the function of animals within a zoo, and how these relate to the zoos goals will place restrictions on the type of environmental enrichment that could be used. However, with some imagination it is possible to develop highly enriched environments for zoo animals, no matter what a zoo's goals are.

7.5 Conclusion

We should always commence our enrichment programme for a species with the determination to provide the best environment possible. Only after we have done this should we then think about the constraints and limitations under which we have to work. If we start by thinking about the constraints and limitations we will almost certainly produce an environment of which the level of enrichment is below that which is achievable. We should only eliminate a good enrichment idea when we are sure that there is no possible way to incorporate it within the animals' enclosure.

Food and Foraging Enrichment 8

The two primary behaviour patterns that determine an individual animal's immediate survival are its ability to avoid predation and its ability to find food. Predator avoidance is usually not a common occurrence and its implementation as an environmental enrichment technique is controversial and illegal in some countries. In contrast, finding food is a common behaviour pattern, often of considerable duration, and utilising it for environmental enrichment is not controversial, unless live food is being offered (Ings *et al.*, 1997). It should be noted that the offering of live prey to carnivores is illegal in many countries (in the UK it would contravene the *Animal Protection Act* 1911 and subsequent amendments) and the ethical position is unclear – the welfare of the predator versus the welfare of the prey species.

8.1 What is Food?

The nutritionist might answer, 'the chemical compounds that a consumer requires for its own bodily maintenance, growth and metabolism'. The ethologist might answer, 'the source of energy that permits short-term survival for animals'. The ecologist might answer, 'the distribution of organic and inorganic resources in time and space, that can be utilised by other organisms for their survival'. The psychologist might answer, albeit flippantly, 'the best source of motivation for enhancing animal learning'. The palatability scientist, 'the source of good health and pleasure'. All of these answers are, of course, correct but perhaps what is interesting is that food means many different things to different specialists and yet it is the totality of these characteristics that has shaped animal (and plant) evolution. Unfortunately, until recent times the importance of looking at all these characteristics has been missed by the scientific community, then in the 1990s scientists started to become interested in the effects of nutrition on behaviour (Young, 1997). In this chapter I intend to look at all aspects of food, feeding and foraging behaviour as they pertain to environmental enrichment and animal welfare.

For the sake of simplicity I have divided animals into those that primarily consume other animals (i.e. carnivores) and those that primarily consume plants (i.e. herbivores). I accept that these are broad and arguable categorisations of animal feeding and foraging strategies. I have applied these two broad categorisations to mammals, birds and certain invertebrates (e.g. octopus) but not to reptiles, amphibians or fish, which I consider separately. It is not my intention in this chapter to describe examples of feeding enrichment for a wide variety of species; instead, I intend to point out the important salient characteristics of feeding and foraging for all species.

8.2 How Animals Forage and Feed

To facilitate the reader's appreciation of the diversity of animal feeding categories and their behavioural consequences, I have followed the work of Seidensticker and Doherty (1996) in using the seminal work of Eisenberg (1981) on classifying mammalian feeding strategies as a guide for feeding enrichment. I believe that Eisenberg's categories are very useful because they make us think about the exact nature of the feeding and foraging behaviour of species. (Although the Order Mammalia contains around 4000 species, Eisenberg has divided them into only 16 feeding categories, a considerable reduction in the quantity of information to be processed.) The important feeding characteristics of carnivores and herbivores that I outline below, should be considered in the light of Eisenberg's work.

At this point I think it would be useful to briefly review the influence of important ecological characteristics of animal species in relation to their feeding and foraging behaviour. The two most important characteristics to us are body size and whether the species feeds primarily on animal or plant material (Illius & Gordon, 1993). As the body size of an animal decreases its metabolic costs multiply, such that a shrew, which weighs around 5 g, has a per-gram metabolic rate 100 times that of an elephant, which weighs 3 833 000 g (Schmidt-Nielsen, 1985). Thus, small animals must consume food that is nutrient dense, whose nutrients are quickly available (i.e. be a carnivore or insectivore) and consume food frequently (e.g. shrews must consume food once every 90 minutes to survive). Conversely, large animals can survive on low quality food whose nutrients can be extracted slowly but usually need to consume food frequently due to the low quality of the food. Among the primates we see this exact trend: gorillas (the largest species) consume almost exclusively plant material; medium-large size primates (e.g. colobines) consume leaves and fruits; medium-small sized primates (e.g. guenons) consume fruits and insects; the smallest size (e.g. bushbabies) are largely insectivorous (Richards, 1985). A behavioural consequence of small body size and high metabolic rate is that such small animals are usually much more behaviourally active than large animals. A behavioural trend also seen in carnivores. Carnivores as an order vary greatly in size but all individuals consume nutrient dense food with quickly available nutrients. Large carnivores, such as lions have the capacity to eat a large quantity of meat at one meal and then survive on this meal for several days. The domestic cat due to its smaller body size (therefore, higher metabolic rate) needs to consume around 12 meals per day (Rainbird, 1988). I am sure you will also perceive the activity difference of these two species; lions are active for only 4 hours in each day whereas domestic cats are active for at least twice this period per day. These relationships between ecology, body size and behaviour are so strong that if a new species of mammal or bird were discovered tomorrow, we would be able to predict its feeding behaviour accurately from knowledge of its body size and whether it is primarily an animal- or plant-consumer.

It is important to remember that body size is an evolutionarily selected adaptation, therefore, if we fail to take it into account when designing feeding regimes for animals we may be causing problems for the animal. Interestingly, it has been found that herbivores in captivity primarily perform oral stereotypies (e.g. tongue rolling) and carnivores locomotor stereotypies (e.g. pacing) that appear to reflect feeding pattern differences (Mason & Mendl, 1997; Carlstead, 1998). The occurrence of these stereotypies is, in part, caused by feeding practices (Carlstead, 1998; Lyons *et al.*, 1997; Terlouw & Lawrence, 1993; Wurbel *et al.*, 1998; Reinhardt & Roberts, 1997; Baxter & Plowman, 2001). Herbivores are fed concentrated food that is consumed rapidly, often in just a few minutes, whereas in the wild they would spend hours ingesting low quality food. Carnivores, on the other hand, are fed meat but it is usually presented in a bowl, therefore, no hunting behaviour can be expressed (Young, 1997).

8.2.1 Carnivores

It is possible to divide the carnivores into two main types, the chasers and the ambushers. It should be noted, however, that many species change between these two strategies depending on environmental conditions. For example, polar bears are able to switch between these two strategies although there are reports of some individuals specialising in one strategy (Stirling, 1990). The sequence of hunting by almost all chasing carnivores follows the following pattern: first, the prey is located by vision, olfaction, or audition, depending on the species; next the predator stealthily approaches the prey (the 'stalk'); when close to the prey the animal chases it (the 'hunt'); and finally, the carnivore kills the prey (Lindburg, 1988). In general, ambushers hide in a location where prey species frequently pass and then usually leap onto the prey (e.g. leopards) or chase it from a very short distance (e.g. tigers) (Kitchener, 1991). Depending on the carnivore species, their prey can move in either two dimensions (e.g. Thompson's gazelles chased by cheetah) or three dimensions (e.g. fish hunted by penguins). In terms of chasers, hunts can be of relatively short duration and distance (e.g. cheetah) or over long distances and periods of time (e.g. African hunting dogs). Furthermore, the predator can hunt solitarily (e.g. the domestic cat) or in a group (e.g. feral dogs). Group hunting animals may also be co-operative hunters (e.g. wolves) or non co-operative hunters (e.g. African hunting dogs; Frame *et al.*, 1979).

The frequency with which carnivores hunt is often related to their body size. Large carnivores and co-operative-hunting carnivores usually feed infrequently (once a day or less), lions feed on average once every 3 days whereas feral domestic cats feed on average 12 times per day (Rainbird, 1988). Of course, feeding frequency is related to prey abundance and other environmental variables. Meat is a nutrient rich source of food and therefore carnivores do not need to spend a great period of time feeding. Given the low basal metabolic rate of large mammals relative to their body size it should not surprise us that large carnivores kill infrequently.

Carnivores can either have a generalist or a specialist body plan. Compare the bodies of pumas (the most widely distributed of cat species) with that of the cheetahs (Kitchener, 1991). The cheetah has many specialist adaptations for its style of hunting, non-retractable claws (increased traction), large nostrils (for breathing in large quantities of air), flexible spine (to increase stride length and, hence, speed), specialised vision (for detecting prey), (for example Caro, 1994). Thus, for chasing carnivores we should be able to highlight the key features of any environmental enrichment device that promotes hunting behaviour:

- In how many dimensions does the prey move?
- What is the average duration and distance of a hunt?
- How many times per day does the species hunt?
- Does the species hunt in groups or solitarily?
- If a group hunter, does it hunt co-operatively?
- Does the species' body plan possess animal specialisations for hunting?
- What sense(s) does the animal use to locate its prey?
- Does the animal use cover to stalk its prey?
- How does the animal capture its prey?
- How does the animal kill its prey?
- How do answers to the above questions vary for different prey species?

We need to take this list of questions and design hunting enrichment that is in concordance with the answers to the above questions. Williams *et al.* (1996) did exactly this when designing hunting enrichment for zoo-housed cheetahs. The cheetahs' prey moves usually only in two dimensions (although, Thompson's gazelle may leap into the air to avoid predation). The average distance of a hunt is between 200 and 400 metres (duration is typically less than 30 seconds). If successful, this species will hunt only once per day. Normally, the species hunts in a solitary manner but occasionally brothers will engage in co-operative hunting. The species' body plan is highly specialised to permit it to run and accelerate very fast (the fastest mammal). Prey is located only by vision (and can only detect prey moving in a horizontal axis) and normally cheetahs climb onto a vantage point such as a termite mound to search for prey. Where cover is available, the animal will make use of it to stalk its prey. Prey is captured by the animal running very fast to become close to the prey and then the cheetah trips its prey up by striking at the prey's legs using a front paw. Cheetahs rarely capture stationary prey due to their low bodyweight. Prey is usually killed by strangulation, the cheetah will then carry its dead prey into a shaded area and often waits up to 30 minutes before commencing to eat its kill (Caro, 1994).

In response to all this information, Williams *et al.* (1996) designed a pulley system that carried a dead rabbit through a zoo-housed cheetahs' enclosure at high speed. The prey was only made available to the cheetahs when they were running, and they were only offered the opportunity to hunt until they had made one successful hunt. A common mistake in some automated hunting enrichment devices is that they allow the animal to choose how often it hunts (Synder, 1977). These systems work on the principle of operant behaviour, i.e. the animal expresses a behaviour (e.g. hunting) and it receives a reward (e.g. food). Many patterns of behaviour can accurately be described as operant (Staddon, 1987), not just the rat in the Skinner Box pressing a lever for a food reward. However, in many scientists' minds operant behaviour and Skinner Boxes are inextricably linked together. The problem is that some animal welfare scientists implement opportunities to perform hunting behaviour as if the animal were in a Skinner Box. The principal difference between operant behaviour in the wild, such as hunting, and operant behaviour in the Skinner Box is that the operant behaviour of wild animals is not always rewarded. Of course, in automated hunting enrichment devices the predator is rewarded on an intermittent schedule, either in number of responses or time; however, such schedules never include the possibility that the animal will not be rewarded that day or even for several days. In the wild, some cheetahs may go several days without a successful hunt, depending on prey availability (Caro, 1994). The problem for care-givers is that it is not usually acceptable to allow an animal to be without food for such a long period of time. However, the problem here is more to do with the ill-thought-out implementation of the reinforcement schedule. Consider the domestic cat, feral members of this species hunt successfully an average of 12 times per day. Given knowledge about their hunting behaviour it should be possible for us to construct an automated (electronically controlled) hunting device. The programming of such a device should use intermittent schedules but with the provision that the animal will be successful once every two hours on average, or that once the animal has received 12 rewards the device will permit more hunting but not reward the animal until the next day. Unfortunately, most examples of such automated hunting devices will continuously reward the animal and it should not surprise us, therefore, that there have been cases of zoo-kept carnivores hunting several hundred times per day (Synder, 1977).

I believe that developing acceptable 'hunting' enrichment devices for ambush predators is a much more complex problem when the animals are housed within a zoo. Consider the polar bear. One of its main hunting strategies in the wild is to find a recently used seal hole in the ice, build a small snow wall to hide behind and then lie flat looking at the hole for up to eight hours. Just before the seal surfaces, it emits some bubbles of carbon dioxide warning the bear of its impending presence. Once the seal surfaces the bear smashes the seal's head against the side of the hole, killing it, and then it drags the body from the water to eat (Stirling, 1990). It would be a relatively simple engineering process to construct simulation ice holes in a polar bear's enclosure which are connected to pipes through which food could be made to appear in the polar bear's enclosure (albeit dead food). However, given that the zoo-going public's most common animal-welfare complaint, albeit misguided, is that the lions are sleeping because they are bored, imagine the public response to a polar bear that spent most of its day staring at an empty hole. As with the case of the lions, one can argue that a public education programme is needed, not compromises in how we enrich the lives of animals. I for one agree with this argument but I also know that effective public education programmes take many years to yield positive results.

The other danger with hunting enrichment in zoos is that you might naturally wish to show this off to the public, as it provides a wonderful education opportunity and, in our polar bear case above, a way to explain what we are doing. Unfortunately, this often results in cues that the food is about to arrive. Either the enrichment is done at set times each day and the animal learns these schedules or the presence of education staff (or a large crowd) become a discriminative stimulus (predicting the arrival of food). Both situations can create animal welfare problems. Lyons *et al.* (1997) found that fixed feeding times were associated with the performance of stereotypic behaviour in zoo-housed carnivores. Fixed feeding times are often associated with aggression in group-fed primates (Bloomsmith & Lambeth, 1995). Examples of hunting enrichment are shown in Figures 8.1–8.4.

8.2.2 Herbivores

The herbivore category includes a wide variety of animal feeding strategies (Table 8.1), however, as was the case with carnivores, we can reduce their feeding and foraging behaviour down to a series of questions that will allow us to design feeding enrichment for them (see below). In this section, for the sake of simplicity, I will define all animals that primarily consume plants as herbivores. Herbivores can be difficult to feed in a species-specific manner for two broad reasons: in the case of farm animal species, they may be food restricted for economic and reproductive reasons (Young, 1999); and the quantity of food consumed by large herbivores may be difficult to provide, e.g. giraffes consume around 66 kg of browse per day in the wild (Pellew, 1984). One common consequence of both these reasons is that the feeding time of the animals is often very short in comparison to their wild-living counterparts (Veasey *et al.*, 1996a). Adult female domestic pigs normally consume their daily food ration in ten minutes (Young, 1993), whereas

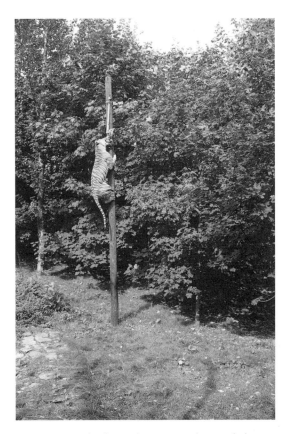

Figure 8.1 A captive tiger using a feeding pole to express hunting behaviour (© Robert J. Young).

their wild counterparts will forage and consume food for up to 75% of the daily period (Young, 1993). Veasey *et al.* (1996a) demonstrated that captive giraffes feed for a considerably shorter period of time in comparison with their wild counterparts. It has been suggested that in both of these cases, short feeding times may be associated with the development of abnormal behaviour (Mason, 1991).

In the case of domestic pigs, food restriction is also an important factor in the development of abnormal behaviour (Appleby & Lawrence, 1987). If, for practical reasons, we must feed some herbivore species on concentrated diets, then we need to give serious consideration as to how we present such diets. Most herbivores are fed from a bowl and a few species are routinely allowed to graze outside, e.g. some farmed sheep races. While it is hygienic and practical to provide feed in a bowl, this completely ignores their evolved feeding and foraging behaviour.

Table 8.1 Mammalian feeding categories.

Feeding Category	Behavioural characteristics
Piscivore and squid eater (fish eaters, e.g. seals, penguins, etc.)	Normally, prey is chased in the water until captured when it is often swallowed whole and while the animal is submerged.
Carnivore (meat eaters, e.g. felids, raptors etc.)	Two methods of hunting exist: (1) the prey species is chased across the terrain (e.g. dogs) or sky (e.g. raptors). (2) the prey species is ambushed, typically by a solitary animal (e.g. leopard). Type 1 hunting may involve long chases (e.g. hunting dogs) or short sprints by the predator (e.g. cheetah). Within a given species all types of hunting behaviour may be used, e.g. polar bears. Type 1 may also involve group hunting (e.g. killer whales) that relies upon group co-operation (e.g. wolves).
Nectarivore (nectar eaters, e.g. humming birds)	The animal moves between patches of flowers, where it feeds usually using a specialised tongue. The animal may have a highly developed spatial memory and the ability to use UV-light to determine on which flowers to forage.
Gummivore (gum eaters, e.g. common marmosets)	The animal moves between trees where it gouges holes in the bark, normally using specialised dentition.
Crustacivore and molluscivore (crustacean and mollusc eater, e.g. walrus)	The animal dives to the bottom of the sea and usually feels for the food using its whiskers, food is then dug up using either fins or mouth.
Myrmecophage (anteaters, e.g. giant anteater)	The animal moves between insect nests which, typically, it breaks open with a claw and then feeds using a long, sticky tongue. Often, these species feed from a nest for only a short period of time and their foraging behaviour could be characterised as harvesting.
Aerial insectivore (flying insect eater, e.g. bats, swallows and swifts)	The animal normally waits until it locates a swarm of insects and then chases them in the air.

Table 8.1 continued

Feeding Category	Behavioural characteristics
Foliage-gleaning insectivore (insect eater, e.g. bushbabies)	The animal may either chase the insects through vegetation or wait until the insects come close and then leap to capture them.
Insectivore – omnivore (e.g. marmosets and tamarins)	Insects or vegetable food are found by moving between patches of vegetation.
Frugivore – omnivore (e.g. Old World primates)	Fruit or vegetable food are found by moving between patches of vegetation.
Frugivore – granivore (e.g. yellow-eyed juncos)	Seeds are either collected when they have fallen to the ground or collected directly from the plant. Normally, the animal moves between vegetation to find food.
Frugivore – herbivore (e.g. ungulates)	Food, usually grasses, is cropped from the ground by grazing.
Herbivore – browser (e.g. goats)	The animal uses specialised dentition to access as much of the plant material as is available.
Herbivore – grazer (e.g. cattle)	Typically, the animal pulls the plant material out of the ground using its tongue and then masticates it.
Planktonivore – nektonivore (plankton and small fish eater, e.g. baleen whales)	The animal filters water through its specialised (baleen) jaw plates to extract plankton, krill and small, shoaling fish.
Sanguivore (blood eater, e.g. vampire bat)	The animal hunts for other animals at night and once encountered, it removes a small quantity of blood using a painless bite.

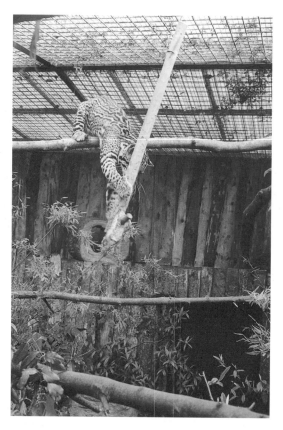

Figure 8.2 A captive ocelot using a swing-pole feeder to 'hunt' for its food (photograph by courtesy of Graham Law ©).

Furthermore, bowl feeding can create a range of behavioural and health problems. The problems usually relate to group-housed animals. In group-housed primates, the bowl can be dominated by one individual who selects only the 'best' food items to consume, such individuals often suffer from diseases that result from an unbalanced diet, e.g. vitamin D deficiency (Young, 1997). Also, spatially highly concentrated food resources, such as bowls and troughs, can result in territorial behaviour as dominant animals defend the food resource (Young, 1997).

Normally, such problems are resolved by designing feeding troughs to protect the feeding individual, e.g. in the case of farmed pigs, single feeding spaces are created along a feeding trough by using solid partitions to create such feeding spaces. The most extreme case of animal protection during feeding is perhaps that of the electronic sow-feeder. In this case, the animal is protected inside a metal cage while it is feeding (Young, 1999). If bowl feeding results in high levels of aggression, some institutions may separate individuals at feeding time, a common

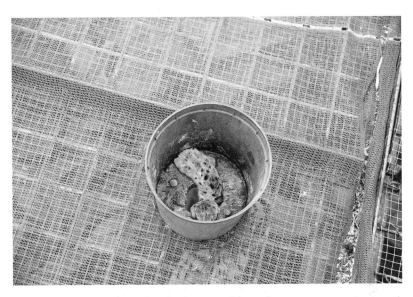

Figure 8.3 A margay using a rooftop feeder (viewed from above); we can see the animal searching with its paws for the food (© Robert J. Young).

practise with laboratory-housed animals where individual daily food intake is often an important variable. Some zoos and laboratories have sought to resolve such problems with primates by training them to feed co-operatively (Desmond & Laule, 1994). All of these solutions are really only attempting to cure the symptoms of the problems that this type of feeding creates rather than resolving the problem. In many species that are housed in a sufficiently large enclosure, the spatial and temporal scattering of their food reduces aggression to normal levels at feeding time and ensures that all individuals receive a balanced diet (for a review of literature see Young, 1997).

The basics for designing a feeding and foraging programme for herbivores can be determined from the answers to the questions below:

- In how many dimensions are food found?
- What is the average distance between food items?
- How many times per day does the animal feed?
- What is the average duration of feeding?
- Does the species feed in groups or solitarily?
- Does the species' body plan possess animal specialisations for feeding?
- What sense(s) does the animal use to locate its food?
- How does the animal process its food?
- How do answers to the above questions vary for different food items?

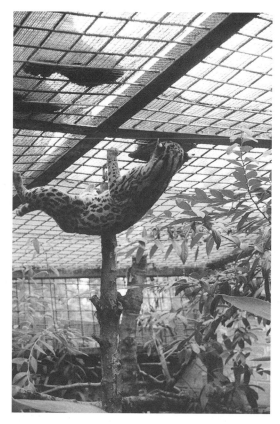

Figure 8.4 A margay using a rooftop feeder (viewed from below); we can see the animal reaching for the food with its paw (© Robert J. Young).

In the case of grazing animals, such as sheep, cattle, rabbits and large ungulates, food is usually found only in two dimensions, i.e. on the ground. One could include in the grazing category, leaf-eating monkeys such as langurs that feed in three dimensions, and grazing primate species such as gelada baboons (Richards, 1985). The average distance between food items in a field of grass can be considered negligible and feeding may occur for one long bout that lasts most of the daylight period, especially because the food consumed is of low nutrient density. These species typically feed in large social groups because they are susceptible to predation in the wild. Typically, these species possess modifications of their digestive system (e.g. a rumen) that permit them to consume large quantities of food, and often have specialised dentition (Illius & Gordon, 1993). Food may be detected by the sense of vision or olfaction, depending on the species. Food is usually pulled from its roots using either tongue, teeth or fingers and placed directly in the mouth for mastication and swallowing. In some species it may also be ruminated. A modification of the above feeding pattern is seen in browsers such as goats and small ungulates, who often possess specialised dentition (e.g. a small dental arc) that permits them to select only certain parts of plants. This feeding modification permits the selection of only nutrient-rich parts of plants, e.g. young shoots or leaves.

The other main style of herbivore are those species that feed on nutrient rich and spatially patchy distributed food. Such species include extractive foragers (e.g. pig species), frugivores (e.g. many primate species) and granivores (e.g. many bird species). These species may find their food in two or three dimensions and typically, their food occurs in small patches that are spatially separated (spatial separation can vary greatly depending on the food source). Typically, these animals spend considerable time looking for food and moving between food patches (i.e. foraging) and relatively little time actually feeding, especially in comparison with grazing animals which spend most of their time feeding. Such species may feed alone or in small groups, exceptions to this occur when food density is very high. These species usually consume a wider range of food items than grazers and tend to have a more generalist body plan. Pigs, for example, have a snout that permits them to dig for food but are equally capable of browsing berries from fruiting bushes (Stolba & Wood-Gush, 1989). Primates posses a hand with five fingers that can manipulate an almost infinite range of food items. Food is usually located by olfaction or vision. In some species we have evidence that animals remember the location of food sources and the timing of food availability, e.g. mountain gorillas (Byrne, 1999).

There are many different methods that exist for enriching the feeding of herbivores, these include: puzzle feeders for manipulative foragers, e.g. primates (Roberts *et al.*, 1999; Novak *et al.*, 1998); foraging devices for extractive foragers, e.g. pigs (Young & Lawrence, 1996; Young *et al.*, 1994); adding hay to a browser's diet, e.g. giraffe (Baxter & Plowman, 2001). Techniques for specifically enriching the lives of ungulates with reference to feeding have been documented by Forthman-Quick (1998) (see Figures 8.5–8.8 for examples).

Finally, sources of information about the toxicity of plants to animal species are listed in Chapter 13.

8.2.3 Reptiles, amphibians and fish

Reptiles, amphibians and fish are physiologically and behaviourally different from mammals and birds (see Schmidt-Nielsen, 1985). Physiologically, this group has a lower metabolic rate than mammals or birds of the same body weight and can, therefore, survive for longer without food. For those interested in environmental enrichment, perhaps the most important difference is the behavioural one (Blake *et al.*, 1998). In comparison with mammals and birds, the behaviour patterns of this group of animals are more like fixed-action patterns (Manning & Dawkins, 1996), i.e. they are more likely to be innate and less modifiable by experience. (I

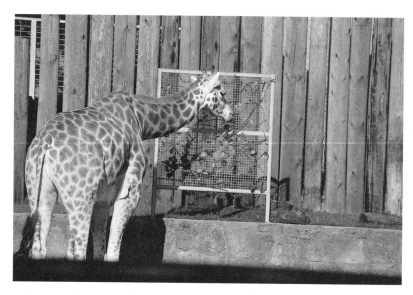

Figure 8.5   A giraffe foraging from a mesh-panel feeder filled with brambles (© Robert J. Young).

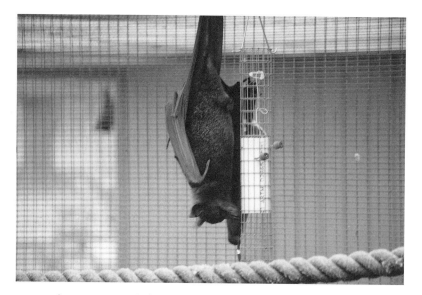

Figure 8.6   A bat using a puzzle feeder; the bat needs to pull out the pins to get the food inside the puzzle (© Robert J. Young).

am certainly not saying that their behavioural repertoire is in place and fixed at birth, just that more of it is in comparison with mammals or birds.) Why is this behavioural difference important? The reason lies in the way that this group of animals is likely to respond to feeding enrichment in comparison with mammals.

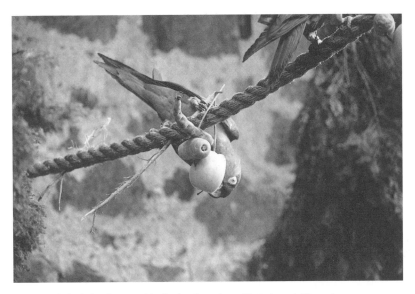

Figure 8.7 A kebab feeder suitable for birds or bats (© Robert J. Young).

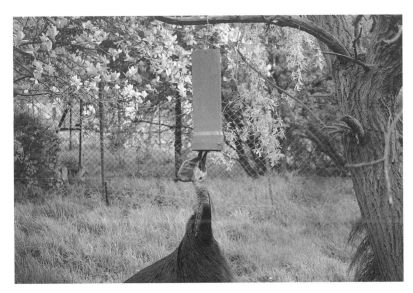

Figure 8.8 A jump feeder for cassowaries; the cassowary needs to jump up and peck at the food inside the tube, thus mimicking its feeding behaviour at bushes in the wild (© Robert J. Young).

I will proceed by way of an example; Shepherdson (1989) found that a mealworm dispenser (a plastic tube with holes drilled in it) attached to the ceiling of an enclosure, from which mealworms fell into the enclosure at unpredictable intervals, was an effective environmental enrichment device for meerkats. The enrichment device stimulated observation and foraging behaviour in the group of meerkats. The same type of enrichment device has been used with insectivorous reptiles whose response to the device was to sit under it and wait for food to fall down (Blake *et al.*, 1998). Thus, their behaviour became fixated and all variation in foraging behaviour disappeared, whereas the meerkats' behaviour became more varied because they were not fixated on the food reward.

All species of animals are susceptible to becoming fixated upon artificial stimuli or artificial reward contingencies, the classic example being that of the super-normal stimulus. Tinbergen (1951), for example, reported a male stickleback becoming highly aggressive when it saw a red postal vehicle passing the window by its aquarium (red being the colour that males use to display to each other). From the scientific literature it is clear that such 'fooling of behavioural systems' is more likely in reptiles, amphibians and fish. I am not saying that the methods we use for mammals and birds are completely inappropriate for these groups of animals but that we need to employ such methods with much greater care and consideration of stimulating fixated behaviour. Remember, environmental enrichment should provide the animal with the opportunity to express motivated behaviour patterns. It is inherent in this that the animal is empowered to make choices; enrichment that results in fixated behaviour has, in my opinion, failed. (Unfortunately, while many mistakes have been made in the enrichment of all animal orders, few of these studies have ever been published, the so called 'file drawer problem' (Rosenthal, 1979), which means that such mistakes will continue to be made.) Feeding enrichment for reptiles, amphibians and fish should concentrate on promoting natural feeding and foraging behaviour. For example, by the provision of live plants for herbivores, the provision of live insects for insectivores and the use of meat trails or artificially moving dead prey, e.g. a dead rat being shaken on a snake feeding pole (for a detailed review see Blake *et al.*, 1998).

8.3 Feeding in General

The two main roles of the animal care-giver are cleaning out the animals' enclosure and feeding the animals. Often, feeding schedules of animals in captivity relate more to care-giver convenience than to what is best for animal welfare. Zoo keepers may feed their animals first thing in the morning in their outside enclosure to facilitate cleaning the indoor enclosure and then feed the animal in the inside enclosure just before the zoo closes, using the hunger the animal has accumulated during the day to motivate it to go inside (Law *et al.*, 1997). Pet owners often feed their cat once before they go to work and then when they return in the early evening.

Does feeding an animal fewer times per day than evolution designed it to feed matter? We might only feed our domestic cat twice a day but if we provide it with enough food is there a problem? This kind of thinking is unfortunately common and totally erroneous. The cat's digestive system is physically designed to consume a certain quantity of food per unit time and overloading the stomach may cause discomfort. (Just imagine consuming all your food in one meal per day.) Much more serious is the fact that the animal's digestive physiology has not evolved to cope with processing such a quantity of food chemicals (e.g. protein) in such a short period of time. The consequence of this can be high levels of alkaline substances in the blood of the cat which in turn cause crystals in the bladder (Young, 1997), a common and serious health problem in domestic cats, so physical well-being is compromised. The provision of only two meals per day, even if they are provided by hunting enrichment, is a low frequency and one which is unlikely to occupy much of the animal's daily time budget. Of course, many domestic cats have cat-flaps and access to potentially unlimited hunting opportunities but a large proportion are now maintained inside the home or in a special enclosure, possibly due in part to the owners' concerns about common diseases of domestic cats such as feline AIDS (McCune, 1997). The thwarting of hunting motivation in felids has been cited as one major cause of the development of abnormal behaviour and stereotypies in felids (Wechsler, 1991; Mason, 1991; Lyons *et al.*, 1997; Mason & Mendl, 1997).

The artificial scheduling of meals for captive animals is associated with a change in the mechanism regulating short-term food consumption (de Castro, 1988). Most wild animals use a hunger mechanism to regulate their food intake, i.e. they eat to a point where their hunger disappears (also called post-prandial regulation). Humans, large carnivores (e.g. lions) and animals fed on an artificial schedule regulate their food intake using a satiety mechanism, i.e. they try to avoid their stomach being so empty that they experience hunger (Le Magnen, 1985). In domestic cats, the physical health risks of this change are well established (see above) but for many other species we do not know what the adverse consequences could be. As is the case with domestic cats, adverse physical consequences might only appear after experiencing years of this feeding method. In the case of farm animal species, they may be slaughtered for food before any physical symptoms appear (most food animals are slaughtered between a few months and three years old); this situation may also apply to many laboratory animals.

It is common for many animal species in the wild to go for long periods of time without food. Nesting male king penguins can be left incubating eggs for several weeks (Charrassin *et al.*, 1998), polar bears in the high Arctic may go months without food, many carnivores do not hunt successfully everyday and wild boar have been observed to lose 30 per cent of their bodyweight during winter (Young, 1993). Most commonly, animals are food restricted due to seasonal changes in the weather that affects their food availability, e.g. black bears in Canada. For animals in captivity, whose wild counterparts undergo seasonal food restriction, should we recreate this period of food restriction (Allen *et al.*, 1996)? The simple answer to this question is that we do not know whether this might benefit physical health. For example, we know that food restriction increases the lifespan of rats (McCay *et al.*, 1939) but this almost certainly causes some degree of suffering, and certainly compromises one of the Five Freedoms (see Chapter 1).

8.4 The Sensory Qualities of Food

In human society, the taste, the appearance, the texture, and the smell of food are considered to be very important characteristics. I think almost everyone in modern human society is revolted by the idea often proffered in science fiction films of humans consuming their daily requirement of nutrients from several tasteless or even tasty pills. It is well known that American astronauts who have been fed the closest to this kind of diet were very jealous of their Soviet or Russian counterparts who ate caviar and steak (Law *et al.*, 1998). To humans food is an important multi-sensory experience, but are such experiences important to animals as well? Undoubtedly, the palatability of food to animals is important: if it were not then pet food companies would not spend so much time and money investigating the subject (Edney, 1988). Although many cynics have suggested that as it is humans who buy the pet food, then, primarily, it has to be attractive to pet owners. It is, of course, true that a hungry animal will eat whatever non-toxic food is placed before it. Cynicism aside, the sensory characteristics of food that are likely to be attractive to animals are taste, visual appearance, texture, smell and auditory properties, e.g. live insect prey.

The importance of taste to animals must be tested under experimental conditions. We cannot say that primates prefer the taste of bananas to apples just because they appear to prefer them. The nutrients contained within each species of fruit are different. Thus, we must look at flavouring experiments to see if species actually do prefer foods on the basis of flavour, i.e. identical food but with different flavours is offered to the animals (Hullar *et al.*, 2001; Narjisse *et al.*, 1997; Baumont, 1996; Provenza, 1995). If possible, we should also investigate the species' ability to perceive different tastes, i.e. which, if any, types of taste receptors does the species possess. There is scientifically credible evidence that certain species prefer certain flavours. Bond and Linburg (1990) showed that captive cheetahs preferred whole carcass feeding to being fed a prepared, soft-textured diet. However, this evidence is not necessarily proof that animals prefer this type of food since the food could have different nutritional content and certainly has different visual, tactile and olfactory sensory input (see below). The preference expressed by an animal may simply result from the influence of maternal diet, especially for mammals (Galef, 1976). Another possibility is genetic propensity to prefer one type of food with an associated flavour; the diet preferences of garter snakes, for example, depend on their environment, coastal or marsh (Arnold, 1981). Furthermore, some species are neophobic (wary of novel food items), e.g. rats (Mitchell *et al.*, 1981). However, we do know that non-coprophagic species avoid eating food contaminated with faecal matter, which obviously relates to physical health (Hutchins *et al.*, 2001), and that many species can learn to avoid toxic food on the basis of its flavour (Provenza, 1996; Provenza, 1995; Provenza *et al.*, 1994). Gorillas in captivity are known to regurgitate and re-ingest sweet food, and it has been suggested that this is because of their strong preference for foods that they cannot obtain in nature, such as cow's milk which is rich in energy (Lukas *et al.*, 1999). It is difficult to prove categorically that the flavour of an animal's food is an important characteristic since the perception of flavour is so strongly influenced by other biological processes. The question of how important taste is to animals is a complex one and depends on things like maternal diet, genetics, etc. Given that animals do display preferences for certain flavours, irrespective of the origin of this preference, we should recognise the importance of flavour in environmental enrichment, especially for animal species that consume many different types of food items, such as primates (Richards, 1985).

Most animal species are either born with a 'template' of how their food looks (or moves) or learn to recognise their food during their juvenile period. Many species of animals form a search image to help them find their food; this is a heightening of sensory reception to prey characteristics (Plaisted & Mackintosh, 1995; Kono *et al.*, 1998; Hanlon *et al.*, 1999). Birds, for example, can have highly developed sensory abilities to detect cryptic insect prey, so developed, in fact, that they do not 'see' non-camouflaged prey. Primate species can recognise by the colour of fruit whether it is ready to be consumed (Barbiers, 1985; Richards, 1985). Kitchener (1999) has reviewed the literature on social learning in felids and in all species he found evidence that juveniles learn to recognise their prey from the food that their mother presents to them. The mother of felids also 'shapes' the hunting behaviour of her offspring by bringing progressively less injured prey for her juveniles to chase and kill. The presentation of inappropriate prey items, by humans, in captivity can result in re-introduced animals hunting inappropriate prey species. Pettifer (1981) found that captive cheetah fed barbary sheep in captivity attempted to kill giraffe calves, African buffalo, zebra and wildebeest upon reintroduction to the wild, despite high abundance of impala, their natural prey. In the case of animals destined for reintroduction, appropriate feeding enrichment may be essential (Young, 1997). Since prey recognition is learnt in many species its importance in feeding behaviour cannot be dismissed.

So far I have only mentioned the visual appearance of the prey species but in the case of carnivores most prey species are also a source of a moving visual stimulus. The fish that penguins feed on provide a strong visual stimulus, one that appears to induce hunting behaviour – in captivity, the feeding of dead fish to penguins presents a number of problems. In many zoos, penguin pools do not contain water currents or they use a biological filtration system, in either case it is difficult to feed the penguins in the water. Some penguins will learn to consume dead fish from a tray but others not, and as a result a number of zoos have resorted to hand-feeding their penguins (personal observation; Stevenson *et al.*, 1994). Another example mentioned already is that of the visual hunting behaviour of cheetahs, which most carnivore keepers solve by throwing their food along the ground at a low level (personal observation). Many pet toys exist, whose main function is to elicit hunting behaviour in domestic cats; a common example being a stick, with a metre of fishing line attached to it and on the end of the line a feather. Thus, for carnivores I believe that food can have important visual properties in terms of movement.

Before consuming food, many species use their sense of touch to identify their food or to orientate their food prior to consumption. Most species of cats use their whiskers to feel the direction of fur or feathers on their prey so that they can orientate it appropriately before commencing the process of consumption. It is believed that the whiskers of many species provide high levels of sensory input about the nature of food (see Young, 1997). A number of species forage actively using their sense of touch, the aye-aye, for example. This species forages percussively by tapping wood and listening for moving insects inside the wood which it then extracts with a long modified digit (Sterling & Povinelli, 1999). Many species of animals have a highly developed sense of touch. Law (1990) describes using pitfall feeders for bears. These are essentially holes in the ground lined with a concrete pipe (to stop the bears from digging) into which food can be dropped and into which bears can reach but not see. Depending on the food offered, a raw egg (in its shell), dog biscuits or raisins, the bear will use different methods to extract the food. The egg is flipped into the palm of the bears paw and extracted without breaking it. Dog biscuits are collected by the bear using a padding motion, this results in the biscuits being trapped between the bear's digits. Soft large foods like fruits are extracted by being speared onto a claw. Walrus use their whiskers to detect prey (crustaceans) hidden under the sea floor (Kastelein & Wiepkema, 1989). The trunk of an elephant contains more than 10 000 muscles, is highly sensitive to touch and is used to select food items (Wiedenmayer, 1998). Thus, even before the food reaches its mouth an animal may have gleaned much information about it.

Once inside the mouth, perhaps in terms of perception taste becomes the most important characteristic. However, we should not dismiss the importance of texture, since texture of food directly relates to its physical properties, e.g. toughness. The physical properties of food that relate to its texture may be important to the species' physical health. Fitch and Fagan (1982) reported that 70% of captive cheetahs fed a soft textured diet (i.e. something equivalent to domestic cat food) developed focal palatine erosion; this condition was caused by maloccluded dentition which resulted in tooth tips making contact with the soft palate each time the mouth was closed. Corruccini and Beecher (1982) found a similar problem with squirrel monkeys fed only on soft diets. In both cases the lack of vigorous tearing and chewing exercise was to blame. In the most extreme example of this type, studies on captive lions have demonstrated that feeding soft diets resulted in weakening of the jaw muscles to such an extent that they could no longer kill their prey (see Young, 1997). Attempts to solve such problems using dog chews or bones have failed since most exotic carnivores will only chew a bone if it has meat attached to it (Fitch & Fagan, 1982). Dental health problems such as these are common in domestic pets and zoo animals. Perhaps they also exist in farm and laboratory animals but no one looks for them or the animals die before such problems can manifest themselves. Finally, in terms of texture, many species of carnivores have mechano-receptors attached to their canines that allow them to adjust their killing bite when they capture prey. It has been suggested that some species of carnivores can 'feel' their way to the killing bite (Kitchener, 1991).

Many species use their sense of smell to detect food, the most famous examples being domestic dogs, domestic pigs and polar bears, all of which have legendary abilities to detect food at great distances. The polar bear is thought to be able to detect the scent of a seal covered in snow at a distance of two miles (Stirling, 1990). Many species use their sense of smell to detect when a food item is ripe and ready for consumption, e.g. primates (Richards, 1985). Once cats have captured their prey, they use their whiskers and their sense of smell to aid location and consumption of their prey, which they cannot see clearly because it is within their minimum focusing distance (Young, 1997).

In terms of the auditory properties of food, I am only going to consider insects in terms of live feeding, since live feeding as already discussed causes a number of ethical and welfare problems. Insectivorous bats, perhaps, rely most on an auditory perception of their food, i.e. the use of reflected sonar signals. Many species of carnivorous animals use audition to locate their prey. Most predator species have particularly acute hearing in the range of the vocalisations emitted by their principal prey species, e.g. owls are sensitive to the ultrasound frequencies that rodents use when communicating. Markowitz *et al.* (1995) have demonstrated how hunting enrichment can be connected to the vocalisation of the prey species without the need to use live prey. In their enrichment a leopard is alerted to the availability of food by the call of a bird (i.e. a recording), the leopard then has an opportunity to undergo simulated hunting behaviour to receive a food reward. This enrichment example is obviously based on associative learning, the leopard learns to associate the bird call with the opportunity to hunt. The performance of this (operant) behaviour may in itself be rewarding to the animal (Hughes & Duncan, 1988). Thus, the amount of sensory input a species receives from its food is potentially enormous. It is something that we should give serious consideration to when developing a diet for a captive animal species.

8.5 Conclusion

In this chapter I have written extensively about the natural foraging and feeding behaviour of animals and related processes. Here I have not been arguing that the wild is best, as this is a concept to which I have many theoretical and practical objections (Veasey *et al.*, 1996b), I would rather that we should draw inspiration and guidelines for enrichment from our understanding of behaviour expressed in the wild. How closely we wish to simulate the wild in order to stimulate captive animals really depends on our reasons for keeping such animals in captivity. Hopefully, the approach I have outlined will encourage people to think about food and its enormous potential to stimulate animals.

Social Environmental Enrichment

The number of ways to enrich the lives of animals is only limited by the ability of humans to think of ideas. However, it is obvious that some forms of enrichment are more effective at improving animal welfare than others. Compare, for example, the influence of social enrichment versus toys on the well-being of laboratory-housed dogs (Hubrecht, 1993). The economic analyses of behaviour (which measure motivational strength) show that social species will work hardest to obtain rewards that restore physiological homeostasis (e.g. food), then social companionship, and then things such as toys (Young, 1999). These laboratory studies are supported by field studies which show that gelada baboons will give up resting time to maintain a constant level of social behaviour when lactating, for example (Dunbar & Dunbar, 1988). This should not surprise us given how vital social behaviour is for survival (Krebs & Davies, 1987).

Animals that live in groups usually do so for two main reasons; to increase the probability of finding food and to avoid predation (Krebs & Davies, 1987). Animals that live a solitary life usually do so due to ecological constraints, e.g. tigers live solitary lives due to the constraints on finding enough food (Kitchener, 1991). However, for many species social living provides more benefits than simply finding food and avoiding predation, it is a major source of stimulation. The social milieu of many species represents a constant source of complex mental stimulation, the complexity and variety of which we could never hope to replace by any form of environmental enrichment (Humphrey, 1976).

9.1 Social Housing of Asocial Species

Many institutions that keep asocial species of animals believe that they experience better welfare if they are housed socially. The social housing of asocial species is most commonly practiced in zoos, where it is common to see large asocial carnivores, such as tigers, leopards and even polar bears housed together in male–female pairs or even in small groups (Mellen *et al.*, 1998). This may be done due to constraints on housing space or due to the belief that it improves animal welfare. However, the social housing of asocial species has received little attention from scientists in terms of its implications for animal welfare. To date the only major study directly investigating this phenomenon was on the social housing of orang-utans in a large group at Singapore Zoo (Poole, 1987). The results of this study suggest an improvement in welfare when orang-utans are socially housed. However, this study can be questioned on a number of methodological issues; for example, the same animals were not observed under social and asocial conditions. Also, it is obvious that we cannot generalise from this single study.

Clearly, more research is need in this area, especially in relation to the social housing of asocial carnivores. Unfortunately, there exists only non-peer-reviewed reports on this subject. For example, Williams, in an unpublished report to the Royal Zoological Society of Scotland, reports that the exploratory and other behaviour patterns of the female polar bear were suppressed when she was housed with a male (see also anecdotes in Meyer-Holzapfel, 1968). In fact, many zoos create refuges for asocial female carnivores when they are housed with a male and the females may spend protracted periods of time in these refuges. While we await further research on this subject I think it would be best not to house asocial species in groups, especially if the species concerned is highly territorial, which is often the case for asocial species. In an inferential study on the influence of factors affecting reproductive success in small exotic felids, the author reported that reproductive success was negatively correlated with increasing group size. The author of this study, therefore, recommended that asocial carnivores should only be pair-housed for the purposes of mating (Mellen, 1991), a situation that occurs for highly aggressive asocial species such as clouded leopards (Law & Tatner, 1998).

9.2 Group Housing of Social Species

The group housing of a social species is perhaps the best method we have to enrich the animals' life. However, it is vitally important to house species in appropriate group structures (Figure 9.1). It has been suggested that the high level of fighting seen between unfamiliar juvenile domestic pigs is, in part, a consequence of an inappropriate group structure (Young, 1993). In general, they are housed together only as a juvenile group, whereas in the wild they would live in a group consisting of several adult females with their offspring. Barnett et al. (1993) found that the introduction of an adult pig to a group of juveniles significantly reduced fighting, a similar result was found for Tonkean macaques (Petit & Thierry, 1994). To take another example, macaque species of primates usually live in a harem system (one male, several females and their offspring). Females are often aggressively competitive between each other and this aggression is actively suppressed by the male, normally by scanning the females periodically and breaking up fights when necessary (Chamove & Anderson, 1989). Thus, the importance of appropriate group

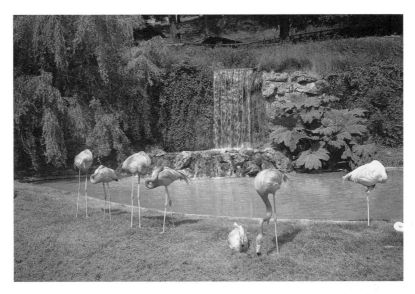

Figure 9.1 A number of animal species, such as flamingos, do not breed when housed in inappropriate group sizes or structures, possibly due to stress (© Robert J. Young).

structure cannot be overstated. However, this does not mean that it is necessary to house animals in exactly the group size and composition that they maintain in the wild. For example, gelada baboons live in mixed-sex groups of up to 200 individuals (Stevens *et al.*, 1992; Richards, 1985; Dunbar, 1983b; Dunbar, 1983a; Dunbar, 1983c). It would be impractical and very expensive for any zoo or laboratory to house these animals in such large group sizes, and probably unnecessary.

Most animals that live in large groups normally, actually spend most of their time with just a few individuals in the group, i.e. in a sub-group. Gelada baboon sub-groups are actually harems consisting of a single male, usually three females and their offspring. Thus, if we needed to house this species it would probably be possible to house it successfully in this sub-group. However, for some species such as flamingos there are critical group sizes below which the animals will not breed, possibly due to the stress of not having sufficient individuals to perform predator avoidance behaviour. Many zoos have reported that flamingos housed in small groups will not breed (Stevens, 1991; Pickering *et al.*, 1992) and in an attempt to solve this problem without increasing group size the zoos have placed mirrors either side of the enclosure (Stevens & Pickett, 1994). The mirrors face each other with the flamingos housed in between, this gives the impression to the flamingos that they are living in a larger group size. Birds and many other species respond to mirrors and videos of conspecifics as if they are real animals (Bloomsmith & Lambeth, 2000; Platt & Novak, 1997). Obviously, this method cannot be used with a species that is highly territorial and responds aggressively to its image, e.g. male gorillas. Recently, some zoos have started to use models of bird species to increase apparent group size (flamingos at Belo Horizonte Zoo, Brazil).

The converse problem of too large group sizes often occurs with farmed animals. Due to economies of scale it is more profitable to produce farmed animals in large group sizes (see Chapter 7). Perhaps the most extreme cases are free-range chickens (for egg production) which may live in groups of up to 10 000 individuals and broiler chickens (bred only for meat production). The greatest problems are seen in free-range laying hens, possibly because they have a greater ability to locomote than broiler hens which grow so fast and heavy that they move relatively little (McLean et al., 2002; Kells et al., 2001; Rauw et al., 1998; Elfadil et al., 1998; Butterworth et al., 2002). In an elegant series of experiments by Grigor et al. (1995a, 1995b, 1995c) he demonstrated that free-range hens are constantly coming into contact with 'strangers' and that they were afraid to pass a stranger. This is not surprising given that they evolved in a harem system of one male, several females and their offspring; this is the social system we see in their closest genetic relative the red jungle fowl from which the domestic hen has been domesticated. Grigor demonstrated it was for this reason that few free-range hens venture outside. In wild animals I know of one analogous situation and that concerns food-provisioned, wild Japanese macaques which live in social groups of more than 1500 individuals compared with the normal maximum group size of 180 (Richards, 1985). Primatologists have describe these groups as being in a constant state of 'anarchy' with high levels of aggression because there are too many individuals for any one individual to recognise (Hill, 1999). Dunbar, for example, has shown that group size is correlated by neocortex size and that the maximum group size for any primate species (in this case humans) should be 150 individuals (Dunbar, 1992; Aiello & Dunbar, 1993; Dunbar, 1995). The Japanese macaque situation is, of course, an artefact of food provisioning but nonetheless demonstrates the potential dangers of too large a group size.

As already mentioned, group composition is important, for example, in most macaque species it is essential that a male is present in the group to minimise inter-female aggression. Thus, the understanding of the roles that different individuals play within a group are of vital importance in implementing social enrichment. Manteca and Deag (1993) have reviewed the potential social roles of animals within groups and demonstrate the importance of such roles in maintaining social stability. The other important component of many social groups is the presence of juveniles and infants. In a number of primate species infants act as a 'social glue' by initiating interactions between adults. For example, chimpanzee infants will often approach and actively solicit social interactions with adults other than their mother (Goodall, 1986). The lack of infants in a social group could, therefore, cause social behaviour problems between adults. This situation is most likely to be a problem within a zoo environment.

With so many species being endangered (in conservation terms), it is now said that species have to compete for access to captive environments (Baliou & Foose, 1996). Many endangered species are now bred so successfully in zoos that most of the population is on contraception. For example, the captive population of golden lion tamarins exceeds more than 100 potential breeding groups but only 15 pairs are allowed to breed each year to prevent over-population. Thus, many groups of golden lion tamarins have no infants, however, the effects of this on this species has not been systematically investigated (De Vleeschouwer *et al.*, 2003). Copenhagen Zoo, Denmark, has dealt with this over-population problem not by using contraception but by euthanasing surplus offspring at the age that they would normally disperse from their parents (Holst, 1997; Holst, 1998). Furthermore, Copenhagen Zoo believe that parenthood is in itself an enriching experience that occupies much of the parents' time but there is no scientific evidence to support this suggestion. However, it is clear from zoo surveys that contraception is not in the best health interests of many species (Hayes *et al.*, 1996). I am not advocating euthanasia as a solution to this problem but it is one solution that is ethically acceptable in Denmark. Animal-welfare problems of course only affect living animals. It is always wise to consider all possible solutions to animal welfare problems.

9.3 Behavioural Development and Socialisation

The importance of mother-rearing of mammals and birds for normal behavioural development cannot be overstated. Animals that are not mother reared do not develop normal social behaviour and react inappropriately to the social signals of their species. Their problems tend to be confounded by the fact that they are reared in isolation and live in this condition into adulthood. Thus, a juvenile primate may react to the threat of an adult with a threat rather than the normal behaviour of submission (Mendl & Newman, 1997).

The most common form of non-mother rearing is hand-rearing (Figure 9.2), which was once widely practised in zoos and laboratories to ensure the survival of animals (van Heezik & Seddon, 2001; Kuehler *et al.*, 1996; Rubin & Michelson, 1994; King & Mellen, 1994). Hand-reared animals show deficits in their social and sexual behaviour, plus, they often perform abnormal behaviours such as body rocking and self-clasping (Mendl & Newman, 1997). Attempts to replace natural mothers with inanimate objects, even those that move, have proved unsuccessful in the development of normal behaviour (Goldfoot, 1977; Mason & Capitanio, 1988). The rearing of animals must be done within the normal range of social relationships, for many species this includes rearing them with individuals other than their mother. Rearing animals in peer groups however, does not necessarily ensure the development of normal behaviour.

In some cases it is unavoidable that the mother cannot rear her infant, for example, she may not have any milk but this does not necessarily mean that we need to use hand-rearing. If we are working with apes we can train them to bottle

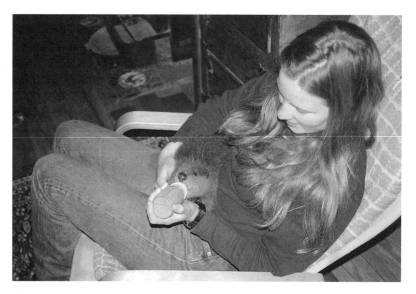

Figure 9.2 An infant beaver being hand-reared and bottle-fed; hand-rearing can result in the development of abnormal social and sexual behaviour (© Robert J. Young).

feed their infants (Zhang *et al.*, 2000; Desmond & Laule, 1994). In other species we might bottle feed the infant but outside of feeding time we can try and maximise contact between an infant and its normal social environment. This may be done by placing the infant directly in that environment or by placing it within that environment inside a cage for protection (Young, 1998). At the very minimum, we should ensure that the animal has contact for a few hours each day with the type of social group that it would normally develop within (Seier & deLange, 1996). In the case of pets, laboratory and farm animals it may be important not only to ensure the development of species normal behaviour that results from maternal rearing but also early socialisation with humans (Krohn *et al.*, 2001; Hubrecht, 1993; McCune, 1997). It is important that species that have close contact with humans are socialised with humans during the 'sensitive period' when they are learning to identify their own species. The proper socialisation of animals with humans results in animals that are less stressed by human contact (which is unavoidable in many animal institutions).

9.4 Rehabilitation and Group Formation

Infant primates, or primates younger than a companion, have been found to be effective in the rehabilitation of older conspecifics that display high levels of abnormal behaviour (often as a consequence of social isolation). Obviously, this method of rehabilitation, depending on the species, can expose the infant to considerable risk of aggression or other types of abuse (Houser *et al.*, 1987; Reinhardt, 1994; Reinhardt, 1991; Reinhardt, 1989; Reinhardt *et al.*, 1988; Reinhardt & Reinhardt, 2000). Thus, the putting together of individuals needs to be done with considerable care and very close monitoring. I will not discuss in detail here the formation of groups of individuals that previously have been isolate housed, such as ex-laboratory primates, because such procedures must only be undertaken in the presence of an expert due to the dangers of severe fighting (Stoinski *et al.*, 2001; Rowden, 2001; Hunter *et al.*, 2001; Johannesson & Sorensen, 2000; Aruguete *et al.*, 1998; Hurst *et al.*, 1996; Alford *et al.*, 1995; Crockett *et al.*, 1994; Barnett *et al.*, 1993; Dunbar & Dunbar, 1981; Houser *et al.*, 1987; Reinhardt *et al.*, 1988; Reinhardt, 1989; Reinhardt, 1991; Reinhardt, 1994; Reinhardt & Roberts, 1997; Reinhardt & Reinhardt, 2000; Reinhardt & Reinhardt, 2002; Young, 1993; and see Chapter 13).

9.5 Managing Social Behaviour

The social life of animals is not always harmonious. Most social species live in a hierarchy and this may be maintained by subordinates avoiding dominants, as is the case with pigs (Young, 1993) or by the dominants reinforcing their position through displays of power, e.g. chimpanzees (Goodall, 1986). There are occasions when certain members of a social group in the wild would avoid other group members. This can occur by simply physically avoiding the same locations as the dominant animal or by hiding from visual contact. It is, therefore, important that we provide opportunities for animals to avoid contact with other group members if they so desire (Rumbaugh *et al.*, 1989; McCune, 1998). These opportunities can be formed by hide boxes, three-dimensional topography or visual barriers in an enclosure, e.g. a curtain of hessian sack strips (Catlow *et al.*, 1998; Figure 9.3). At Edinburgh Zoo visual barriers are used successfully to reduce the intimidation of females and juveniles by adult males in Diana monkeys (Young, 1998). An obvious but important point is not to create visual barriers for species that live in essentially two-dimensional environments (Chamove & Anderson, 1989). It is also important that enclosures that have two areas, an inside and outside area, have at least two exits, for example. Some experienced animal care-givers have suggested that the enclosures for social housing animals should have rounded corners (Maple & Perkin, 1996), not the traditional square ones, as this prevents the cornering of an animal that is the target of aggression.

Social behaviour of animals can of course be managed by human care-givers. One form of management is behavioural modification (Burks *et al.*, 2001). A number of institutions have modified the behaviour of large dangerous animals through positive reinforcement (Figure 9.4). Drills have been rewarded positively for expressing affiliative behaviour, such as grooming (Cox, 1987). In a number

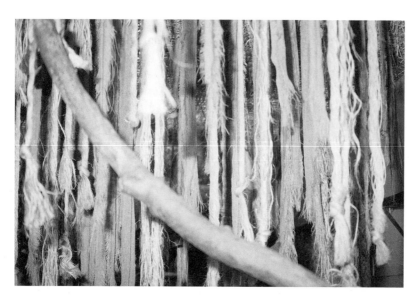

Figure 9.3 A visual screen created inside a primate enclosure using hessian sacking to allow group members to avoid visual threats from aggressive group members without impeding their access to the enclosure area (© Robert J. Young).

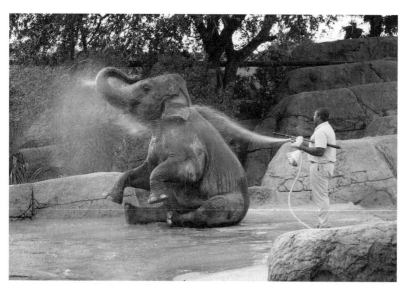

Figure 9.4 An elephant complying with an animal-training procedure; it is possible, using operant conditioning, to modify social behaviour (© Robert J. Young).

of species, individuals have been trained to feed co-operatively (Desmond & Laule, 1994). Finally, animals can be trained to desist from what humans perceive to be anti-social behaviour. I would, however, warn against too much interference in animals' social interactions. Most species have evolved methods of regulating social behaviour (Krebs & Davies, 1987) and if we create appropriate groups housed in appropriate enclosures then we should not need to manage their social behaviour. Catlow *et al.* (1998) have described this as 'hands-off' enrichment and is based on their experience of managing a multi-male multi-female chimpanzee group. In the past, the males in the group were isolated from each other at night because of the (still) widespread fear of fatal fighting between males (de Waal, 1983; Goodall, 1986; Alford *et al.*, 1995). However, it was noted that most mornings when the males were introduced to each other the probability of a fight was high; this situation continued for many years until Catlow *et al.* (1998) started to manage the group. They knew that fatal fighting should not evolve in a species and that all social species have methods of regulating social behaviour, especially aggression. Catlow *et al.* (1998) then stopped locking the males apart at night and the probabilities of any fights quickly became very low. Fights are a natural part of nearly all social species' lives and we should only become concerned when such fights occur in the wrong social structure or a badly designed enclosure. In fact, for some species, fights are necessary to induce reproductive activity, e.g. Egyptian spiny-tailed lizards (Alberts, 1994), or to create a stable dominance hierarchy that will ultimately lead to less aggression (Krebs & Davies, 1987). It is all too tempting to interfere in the fights of animals because their occurrence distresses humans. This can create more problems than it resolves, as aggressive animals are often removed from the social group for a period of time and then re-introduced without the stimulus causing the aggression being removed. Thus, the aggression recommences often with a higher level of intensity. If this cycle is repeated it is possible to create an animal that is so aggressive that it cannot be re-introduced to its social group (Catlow *et al.*, 1998). We then have the huge welfare problem of a social animal that is being solitary housed.

9.6 Solitary Housing of Social Species

There are cases in which isolate-housing a social species is unavoidable. Undoubtedly, the group of animals that is most commonly isolated-housed is pets. Many species of pets are extremely social, the domestic dog being the prime example. Although, the public apparently become very upset at the idea of isolate-housing laboratory animals, they rarely consider the plight of their own pet (see Chapter 7). Separation anxiety in dogs is one of the most common behavioural problems that domestic dogs demonstrate (Overall *et al.*, 2001; Flannigan & Dodman, 2001; Wells & Hepper, 2000b; Simpson, 2000; Turner, 1997; Appleby, 1993; Voith & Borchelt, 1985). Thus, the scale of the problem in pets should not be under estimated; however, at the moment we have relatively little information about the psychological well-being of companion animals. The physical abuse of animals is something that is prosecutable in the UK under the *Protection of Animals Act* (1911 and subsequent amendments) but no such legally enforceable protection exists for psychological suffering. I must point out that in the UK isolate-housing of any social laboratory species is rarely used and needs to be specifically justified to the Home Office under the *Animal (Scientific Procedures, Act* (1986). I have personally visited many animal laboratories in the UK and have never seen social species isolate-housed. The other common cause of isolate-housing of a social species occurs in zoos when it is not possible to obtain a new mate for an animal whose mate has died.

An example of a species that suffers this problem is gorillas. There are around the world a number of male gorillas living a solitary life because it is not possible to find them a mate. The problem is caused by the fact that gorillas live in a harem system (one male and several females) but their birth : sex ratio is 1 : 1. Thus, there are many surplus males in the captive population (and for that matter the wild population). In such harem species a number of attempts have been made at forming bachelor groups of males with mixed success (Alford *et al.*, 1995; Patton *et al.*, 2001; Stoinski *et al.*, 2001). Unfortunately, few zoos wish to risk the adverse publicity when such experiments go wrong and so the real level of success is unknown. Also for many long-lived species these bachelor group experiments have not existed long enough to make a proper assessment of their success, the gorillas being a case in point. Grouping young male gorillas together is likely to be successful during the whole of their prolonged juvenile period (15 years) as they live in their natal group until this age. However, as the males become adults and wish to disperse, the success of these bachelor groups really will be tested.

9.7 The Value of Human–Animal Contact

There are a number of potential solutions to the solitary housing of animal species when solitary housing is unavoidable. Perhaps the most common solution and the solution that people are most unaware of is human contact (Figure 9.5). For many species human contact can, to a degree, substitute for contact of conspecifics. Most research into the human–animal bond has focussed on the therapeutic effects that animals have on human physical and mental health (Bauman *et al.*, 2001; Bernstein *et al.*, 2000; Headey, 1999; Brodie & Biley, 1999; Levoy, 1998; Rowan & Beck, 1994; Brodie, 1981; Davis & Balfour, 1992). One exception being Poole (1998) who has widely written about the value of the human–animal bond to the animal. Bayne *et al.* (1993) demonstrated that only six minutes per week of human contact was enough to significantly reduce abnormal behaviour in rhesus macaques. It has been shown that positive human–animal interaction is associated with reproductive success and a reduction in stress in small exotic felids (Mellen,

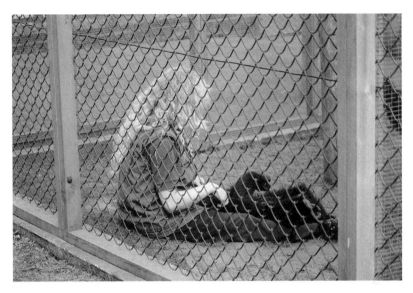

Figure 9.5 Interaction between a care-giver and a primate; here, the keeper is grooming a gibbon (© Robert J. Young).

1991), domestic felids (McCune, 1997), and farm animal species (Hemsworth & Gonyou, 1997; Hemsworth & Barnett, 1987; Hemsworth *et al.*, 2000; Pedersen *et al.*, 1998). In the case of farm animals, however, it is consistency in behaviour of the stockhand that has proven to be the critical factor in the level of animal welfare experienced (the more consistent the stockhand's behaviour the better the animals' welfare). However, even two hours per day of conspecific contact is not enough for the development of fully normal social behaviour in rhesus monkey infants (Goldfoot, 1977).

The exact welfare plight of solitary-housed pets is unknown but the contact of their human care-givers undoubtedly alleviates some of their welfare problems. In English we have a verb to describe human–animal interaction, petting. On farms, in homes, zoos, and laboratories this unconscious interaction may also take place through the animal care-givers' petting or animal training. A reduction in the petting of domestic cats has been associated with an increase in stress levels (McCune, 1997). I believe that the daily training of a solitary-housed social species is very important to its welfare because it ensures daily social contact. (It is interesting to note that in human prisons solitary confinement is often used as the most extreme form of punishment.) Animal training in zoos and laboratories is also used to facilitate veterinary procedures (Bloomsmith *et al.*, 1998; Brown & Loskutoff, 1998; Desmond & Laule, 1994; Zhang *et al.*, 2000) which in itself improves animal welfare. However, for a solitary-housed species I believe that social contact is equally important. It has been reported that training reduces abnormal behaviour in captive stellar Sealions (Kastelein & Wiepkema, 1988) but further experiments are needed to disentangle the effects of training from human contact.

9.8 The Value of Contraspecific Contact

One can question whether contraspecific contact actually improves welfare; although not systematically studied, many scientists have used non-conspecific companions in social isolation experiments. For example, Hsia and Woodgush (1984) isolate-housed domestic pigs with a sheep because their casual observations had shown that pigs did not become stressed under such conditions, whereas they did when housed without any companionship. In the horse racing industry, some trainers house their horses with a goat in order to provide companionship. It should be noted that even in the wild some species form mixed groups (Buchanan-Smith & Hardie, 1997). Goodall (1986) has reported that young chimpanzees will often actively engage baboons in social play and not solely for food or anti-predator benefits. Humans often engage their pets in play behaviour, which appears to be highly stimulating for both parties and has been well documented in dogs (Rooney & Bradshaw, 2002; Rooney et al., 2000). Play behaviour is considered a desirable behaviour and has been used as a measure of animal welfare (Chapter 3). In laboratories, human interactions with dogs have been shown to be an important source of stimulation (Hubrecht, 1993) and many laboratories include it as part of their daily enrichment routine for dogs and cats (personal observation; Loveridge, 1998; McCune, 1997).

Of course, if an animal has been hand-reared by humans to the degree that it is socially and sexually imprinted on humans it may 'regard' humans as its own species (Aengus & Millam, 1999). In fact, it is often reported in human–parrot relationships that when the human owner dies the animal develops abnormal behaviour such as self feather plucking (Evans, 2001; Lantermann, 1997). The most famous long-term relationship between a human and an animal is that of the relationship between a mahoot (traditional elephant trainer) and an Asian elephant (Hart, 1994). In fact, the changes in the socio-economic situations of many Asian countries has resulted in a breakdown in this long-term relationship (traditionally, a boy of five years old is put with an elephant of the same age and they spend their lives working together) and this has been blamed for the increase in behavioural problems, such as aggression towards humans, with Asian elephants (Hart, 1994).

9.9 Limited Physical Contact

Crocket et al.(1998) have investigated the use of limited physical contact between solitary-housed primates. After a series of experiments, Crockett discovered that the best system was one in which both participants could control whether they engaged in physical contact with another individual. To facilitate this she set up a row of primate cages, each of which had a solid door that the occupant could open. The primate was then separated by a series of bars through which it could reach to touch and groom a neighbour, but only if the neighbour also opened its door. This set-up proved to be extremely successful in promoting socio-physical interactions, such as grooming, in macaque species. The ability of the macaques to control the opening of the door provided the animals with the ability to control their social environment, albeit in a limited manner. It is important for us to remember that many species in the wild can control their social interactions by avoiding or actively soliciting interactions.

9.10 Visual, Auditory and Olfactory Contact

Many laboratories that house social animals are designed so that solitary housed animals can see each other, this can be through bars or windows (McCune, 1997; Loveridge, 1998). The degree of social contact can be enhanced by creating channels for auditory and olfactory communication. A co-operative toy could be installed between different enclosures to promote social interactions, e.g. tug-of-war toys. The most important feature of such environments is that the animals can control the level of social contact they experience.

A number of animal species respond to televised images of conspecifics as if they were real animals (Lea & Dittrich, 1999; Anderson, 1999; Bloomsmith & Lambeth, 2000; Platt & Novak, 1997; Eddy et al., 1996). This offers another opportunity to provide some social contact or stimulation for solitary-housed animals. The two main options we have are to show the behaviour of conspecific animals relayed live or to show videos (i.e. pre-recorded behaviour) of conspecific animals. The first option, if available, is clearly more practical as it does not need hours and hours of video tape (in fact, it only requires a camera, a television and a connecting cable). I would recommend in this situation that the animal has the option to switch the television off if it so desires. A number of institutions have experimented with showing live television to animals as a form of enrichment but it would appear that animals habituate to such visual stimuli rapidly, if they ever look at it at all. (The most amusing example I heard was of a zoo that was showing pornographic movies to gorillas in the hope that it would stimulate them to mate!) A similar approach to showing the behaviour of a live conspecific is to reflect an animal image through a series of mirrors, the last image being one that our target animal can see (perhaps a cheaper and more robust solution in some cases).

One of the cheapest non-animal or human companionship solutions that has been used with a number of species is the use of mirrors (Brent & Stone, 1996; Lambeth & Bloomsmith, 1992). Obviously, mirrors will not work as companions with animals that can recognise themselves in mirrors (i.e. the great apes and dolphins) or animals that respond aggressively towards mirrors. In a series of

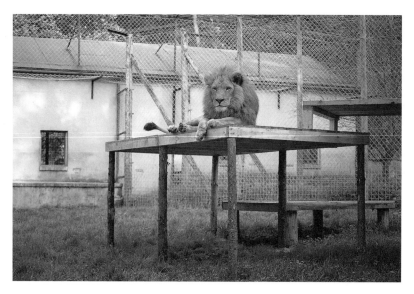

Figure 9.6 Big cats, such as lions, appear to enjoy resting on a raised platform. (Photograph courtesy of Simon Wakefield ©).

experiments Mills *et al.* (personal communication) demonstrated that mirrors were highly effective in reducing the performance of stereotypies (an indicator of poor animal welfare) in solitary-housed horses. However, the long-term efficacy of mirrors in alleviating problems of solitary housing has not been tested. It also unclear how mirrors alleviate the abnormal behaviour of horses: do they substitute for companionship, i.e. the horse reacts as if another horse is present, or are they merely a source of visual stimulation?

In the absence of being able to provide any visual social stimuli a number of animals appear to be motivated to see beyond the walls of their enclosure. Primates and pigs (Matthews & Ladewig, 1994; Anderson, 1998) will work for the opportunity to see the outside world or into an empty pen. Obviously, we do not know what kind of benefits, if any, they derive from this (but see Chapter 10). Interestingly, it has been shown that providing horses with several windows (i.e. visual horizons) reduces the performance of abnormal behaviour (Cooper *et al.*, 2000). It has been shown that large captive felids usually select a resting place from where they can view the environment around their enclosure (Lyons *et al.*, 1997; Figure 9.6).

9.11 Conclusion

The provision of the correct social environment can be the source of endless stimulation for social animal species. It is important, therefore, to recreate natural group structures, composition, and sizes whenever possible; however, we must be aware that there is an interaction between these factors and the captive environment. For example, if we place food in a small pile within an enclosure we may cause territorial aggression (Lowen & Dunbar, 1994; Nijman & Heuts, 2000) and a reduction in the number of animals that can be safely held within that enclosure. In the case where animals cannot be group-housed a number of other methods of stimulating natural social behaviour have been proven to be better than simple isolation rearing. However, none of these techniques solicits the full range of species-specific social behaviour, just as non-mother rearing never results in full behavioural competency of juveniles. In the case of asocial species we must not fool ourselves into believing that what they really want is to be sociable!

Housing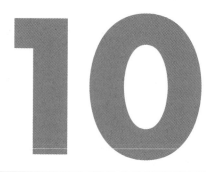

The environment in which an animal is contained is composed of two primary parts, the actual animal enclosure, sometimes referred to as the intrinsic or micro-environment, and the area surrounding the enclosure, sometimes referred to as the extrinsic or macro-environment. Both parts of the animal's environment have an influence on the animal's welfare and can be designed to have enriching properties. In this section I will first consider the animal's enclosure and second the area surrounding the enclosure.

10.1 Looking at Species and Housing Levels

After social behaviour is considered, perhaps the next most important features of an animal's environment are the housing and the 'furniture' contained within it. With the huge number of different species housed in captivity it is difficult to know where to start, however, Seidensticker and Forthman (1998) have provided us with a useful way of reducing this complex problem to a manageable size. They have suggested that we follow the work of Eisenberg (1981) on life histories and divide animals into groups that live on different substrate types. The list of substrate types described by Eisenberg (1981) include:

- fossorial, i.e. adapted for digging, e.g. mole rats;
- semifossorial, i.e. adapted both for digging and terrestrial living, e.g. badgers;
- aquatic, i.e. living solely within water, e.g. whale and fish species;
- semiaquatic, i.e. living both in the water and terrestrially, e.g. seal and penguin species;
- volant, i.e. animals adapted for flying or gliding, e.g. bats and many bird species;
- terrestrial, i.e. adapted for living on land, e.g. most ungulate species;
- scansorial, i.e. adapted for climbing, e.g. many primate species;
- arboreal, i.e. adapted for living in trees, e.g. many bird and primate species.

10.2 A Substrate Approach to Housing

Recognising which type of substrate an animal primarily exists on should provide us with an excellent starting point to think about its housing requirements. It should also help us to focus in on the question of utilisable space. What I mean by this is that although we may provide an animal with an enclosure of 30 000 m², this is not the amount of space necessarily available for the animal to utilise. While it is obvious that if the enclosure of a dolphin contains much terrestrial substrate this area must be discounted in terms of the amount of utilisable space, it is not always so obvious for other species. For example, many species of primate are strictly arboreal (that is, they never willingly come to the ground), therefore, their utilisable space within an enclosure must be calculated only in terms of arboreal space. Unfortunately, all too often this aspect of the animal's environment is a secondary consideration to the total size of the enclosure. I have seen a number of large primate enclosures for strictly arboreal species that have a single tree in the centre, i.e. effectively the animals live on a small island. In some cases I have seen zoos try to increase utilisable space by forcing an animal to use a substrate for which it is not evolved. For example, some zoos will throw the food of strictly arboreal species onto the floor and then claim that they have doubled the utilisable space of the enclosure. Animals have evolved to live on specific substrates in response to predation pressure and food availability (Krebs & Davies, 1987; Hill & Dunbar, 1998). Clearly then, forcing a species onto an 'unnatural' substrate is unlikely to be good for its welfare. Carlstead *et al.* (1993) found that even the wrong type of floor substrate, one with which a small exotic cat (leopard cat) could not blend using its natural coat camouflage, was stressful.

We need to think about the space that an animal lives in as being three dimensional, even for large ungulates, like elephants, that appear to live only within a two-dimensional domain. Few terrestrial animals live in the completely flat world of the 'football pitch' type of zoo enclosures that were popular in the 1960s, 1970s and still exist in some zoos today (Bostock, 1993). Most terrestrial species evolved within terrain that has undulating topography and they often make use of such features. Many species will use a high spot to look for prey, cheetah, for example (Caro, 1994). Even for species that make no use of terrain topography, the sky above them might be very important. Mongoose species such as meerkats (semi-fossorial species) live in an environment almost totally devoid of overhead cover, and this allows them to scan for aerial predators such as hawks (Moran, 1984; Clutton-Brock *et al.*, 1999a; Manser, 1999; Clutton-Brock *et al.*, 1999b). Therefore, the provision of trees or other forms of cover in their enclosure is unlikely to improve their welfare – the very opposite might, in fact, be true. Thus, knowledge of how a species uses its substrate, and the juxtaposition of this substrate to others is of vital importance.

I am deliberately not going to discuss in depth the ongoing and controversial subject of how much space a species requires in captivity. I will reiterate what I have said earlier that beyond a certain minimum amount of space (i.e. quantity of space) the thing that is important is the quality of space (see Chapters 1 and 3; de Waal, 1989). As has been pointed out to me many times by Law (personal communications), the more space you give an animal the greater ability you have to provide things that enrich the animal's life (Shepherdson, 1999). Whether science will be able to answer the question of what is the minimum amount of space a species requires in captivity to experience good animal welfare remains to be seen. Undoubtedly, Law's answer is correct – give the species as much space as possible so long as you utilise this space to enrich the animal's life. Obviously, if we know that a small rodent species in the wild has a maximum area of $1000\,m^2$ then it is pointless to exceed this size, so long as the animal is being provided with the correct kind of utilisable space.

10.3 A Bottom-up Approach to Animal Housing

In terms of thinking about the space for a species, I suggest that it is best to start with the floor or bottom of an enclosure and work upwards. While we primarily need to focus on the needs of the species to be housed within the enclosure, we must also consider the needs of the human care-giver cleaning the enclosure, for example, and health and safety regulations (Rosenthal & Xanten, 1996). At each vertical level within an enclosure we need to think how an animal interacts in that 'level' (altitude if you prefer) of space. The bottom of an enclosure is always a substrate through which the animal can go no further down, even if it is a fossorial species. Although it is possible to house such species without a bottom limit, this makes species management very difficult; many zoos have experience of unmanageable fossorial and semifossorial species in such enclosures.

Perhaps our first question should be, does the species use the bottom substrate in its natural environment? For example, a strictly arboreal species has the forest floor as its bottom substrate but never uses it. In this case, one could argue that the lowest branch is the species bottom substrate (Hebert & Bard, 2000). However, as all environments have an ultimate 'bottom' substrate it is useful to think in these terms. Thus, for strictly arboreal species we should not give great attention to the bottom substrate, except perhaps to colour it the same as in the wild to avoid reflected light induced stress problems (Carlstead et al., 1993). Some institutions, such as zoos, might be using a naturalistic exhibit, in which case it is justifiable to make the bottom substrate look natural, but only if this is not at the expense of providing high quality utilisable space. In fact, housing strictly terrestrial and arboreal species that are compatible in the same enclosure might be the best use of this space (Thomas & Maruska, 1996).

If our animal species does use the bottom substrate, we need to consider why and how the animal uses it. Terrestrial animals like domestic pigs carry out nearly all their highly motivated patterns of behaviour on the bottom substrate. They forage in it by rooting with their snout, they sleep on it, they dig birthing nests in it, they socialise with conspecifics on it etc. (Beattie *et al.*, 2001; Olsen *et al.*, 2000; Burne *et al.*, 2000; Arey & Maw, 1995; Beattie *et al.*, 1998; Haskell & Hutson, 1996). Clearly, the bottom substrate needs to have a number of physical properties. It needs to be strong enough to support the weight of the animal(s) as it moves around and it needs to be excavatable. Stolba and Wood-Gush (Stolba & Wood-Gush, 1984; Stolba & Wood-Gush, 1989) investigated the housing needs of domestic pigs by studying their behaviour when released into a semi-natural environment. Through this method they were able to identify important characteristics of any domestic pig housing as outlined above. They also found that domestic pigs, and probably most animal species, use different parts of their environment for different behaviours, e.g. foraging versus defecating. Whilst the type of study carried out by Stolba and Wood-Gush (1989) is rare, the basic way that many species interact with their bottom substrate is known. It is of course worth pointing out that bottom substrates vary in their physical properties in the natural environment and the captive environment should reflect this. For example, the bottom substrate for beluga whales is the ocean floor which may be sandy, rocky etc. During the summer, beluga whales migrate to shallow rocky areas against which to rub their skin and thereby facilitate their moult (O'Corry-Crowe *et al.*, 1997). Thus, the bottom substrate not only has physical properties but the species' need for such properties can change over the course of a year.

For many species the bottom substrate also assists in the species' predator avoidance. For example, many species possess camouflage markings that blend with the bottom (or other) substrate. Carlstead *et al.*, (1993) demonstrated that the failure to take this into consideration caused considerable stress in zoo-housed leopard cats. Although we do not have scientific evidence on other species we do know that camouflage markings evolved in response to predation pressure (Krebs & Davies, 1987). Most fish species are darker on their dorsal (top) side so that predators looking down on them find it more difficult to distinguish them from the bottom; conversely, they are lighter on their ventral (bottom) side to help blend in with the brighter light above. Therefore, substrate patterning and colouration is likely to be of importance to all species that use camouflage markings.

Finally, we come to the choice of substrates. It is often not possible to use natural substrates because they are not available or practical in a captive setting. However, above we have a set of criteria that should help us to select the most appropriate substrates for each species. Remember, it is the physical properties of a substrate that are important not the substrate *per se*. Practical considerations are also very important in substrate choice. For example, straw and forest bark might both make suitable substrates for a semi-arboreal primate species but forest bark is more hygienic and requires less cleaning effort (Chamove *et al.*, 1982; Chamove &

Anderson, 1989; Ludes-Fraulob & Anderson, 1999). Of course, one should consider the possibility that a substrate can cause irritation or other forms of distress to a species; for example, woodchips are known to affect the olfactory perception of rabbits adversely (Austen, 1994). The final practical consideration is one of local climate when animals are not housed in climate controlled rooms. For example, forest bark could be an excellent substrate in the UK with its mild temperatures and relatively damp climate but this substrate would not be so useful in the dry and arid climate of Australia due to the production of dust particles that could affect animal and human health. It is, of course, possible to conduct choice tests on substrate preference (Mills *et al.*, 2000; Beattie *et al.*, 1998) but such tests only reveal which is the least aversive substrate (Duncan, 1978).

The final point of importance in relation to a terrestrial bottom substrate is how 'soft' the substrate appears to be. The larger the animal species the more important the softness of the bottom substrate. This is because body volume and skin surface area do not increase in direct proportion to one another. As the body volume and hence body weight increases, the amount of relative surface area decreases by the power of 2/3 (Schmidt-Nielsen, 1985). Thus, large animals have a high contact pressure to lying area ratio, as discussed by Nilsson (1992) for dairy cattle. (For a review of the importance of considering the physical properties of materials in animals' enclosures, see Heidbrink, (1997).)

The next question to be asked is what the space between the bottom substrate and the top of the enclosure should be filled with. The possible answers are:

- only air;
- air penetrated by structures such as trees;
- only water;
- water penetrated by structures such as rocks;
- only soil;
- soil penetrated by structures such as plant roots.

As with the bottom substrate we need to ask ourselves how a particular species utilises this level in the enclosure. Do they forage here, build nests here, use this level to escape from predators, use this area for movement? As before, we need to think about the properties of the substrates we offer. For example, most arboreal species of primates climb on branches that move under their weight and this requires of the animal greater strength and hand-eye co-ordination than static branches (O'Neill *et al.*, 1991; Wormell & Brayshaw, 2000; Stafford *et al.*, 1994; Hebert & Bard, 2000; McKenzie *et al.*, 1986) (see Chapter 11). Such physical properties of the animal's environment are essential in maintaining the animal's physical fitness. One criticism that has been raised at zoos in the past is that the animals they rear may have low muscle to body weight ratios, and may even be overweight (Schwitzer & Kaumanns, 2001; Weinsier *et al.*, 1998; Terranova & Coffman, 1997). It is interesting to note that physical exercise in humans is associated with both physiological and psychological well-being (Todd *et al.*, 1992; Salmon, 2001; Oweis & Spinks, 2001; Motl *et al.*, 2000; Hassmen *et al.*, 2000; Berger, 1996; Weyerer & Kupfer, 1994). Certainly, a number of environmental enrichment studies claim increased exercise as a benefit (Henderson & Waran, 2001; Markowitz *et al.*, 1995; Williams *et al.*, 1996). The physiological changes associated with exercise are the same in most mammal species, therefore, there is also the possibility that exercising mammals also obtain psychological benefits from exercise. Animals deprived of exercise for some time show a rebound effect (i.e. perform much exercise) when they have the opportunity (Houpt *et al.*, 2001; Harri *et al.*, 1999). Exercise has been demonstrated to be of benefit to humans with psychological problems (Chamove, 1986) and in animals with psychological disturbances (Takeuchi *et al.*, 2000).

At the very basic level, an animal's environment should challenge the animal's body to maintain its physical strength. If an animal cannot use its normal mode of locomotion then clearly there is something wrong in the environment's design. It has been observed that some bird species lack the ability to fly properly due to the lack of opportunity to fly and the consequent atrophy of flight muscles. I have personally seen primates that cannot climb on moving branches due to a lifetime of being housed on static branches; this was also a problem in the original golden lion tamarin reintroduction project (Tudge, 1992). Obviously, when one has an extreme case like the one described before, it is necessary gradually to physically challenge the animal's body until it regains full fitness and hand-eye co-ordination. Obviously, certain types of animal locomotion may require a minimum space size; for example, the porpoising locomotion of gentoo penguins requires a large pool, cheetahs require a large enclosure to run at full speed, and birds require a sufficiently large and unobstructed space to fly. It is possible, of course, for some species to use devices such as running wheels to promote exercise (Chapillon *et al.*, 1999; Harri *et al.*, 1999; Sherwin, 1998; Kingston & Hoffman-Goetz, 1996). As a comment, animals often prefer not to perform these types of energy-demanding forms of locomotion and will only do so if stimulated to do so. In the case of the cheetah this requires appropriate visual stimulation (Williams *et al.*, 1996) and for birds this might mean distributing resources such as food and water in a manner that forces birds to fly between them. In the past, many zoos have invested in large enclosures for ungulates, such as giraffes, only to discover that they never move far from water, food and shelter resources (Veasey *et al.*, 1996a). Thus, resources should be scattered around the enclosure of the animal to promote locomotion. However, this does not necessarily mean converting the whole enclosure into a foraging patch. It means if the animal naturally discovers its food in clumps then its food should be in clumps around the enclosure. Remember, few animals are surrounded by all the resources they need in the wild.

The health and safety issues discussed for the bottom substrate environment are of course applicable to this environment. Another consideration is the quality of the air, water or soil. One should consider how many air or water changes per hour or soil changes per time period are necessary to maintain a high quality environment in which the risk of pathogen spreading is minimised. For laboratory animals the minimum (and maximum) number of such substrate changes per hour are often legal requirements and these must be adhered to, e.g. see Home Office regulations in the UK (Chapter 13). Different systems of air, water and soil quality control can affect the way in which a species is managed. Take the aquatic environment, which can be kept safe from pathogens using chemicals (e.g. chlorinating the water) or using biological filters (Boness, 1996). The use of chemicals can have adverse effects on animals' physical health but provides opportunities for feeding animals in the water. Biofilters do not expose animals to chemical risks but often cannot cope with a high input of dead organic matter (i.e. food), thus, the animals cannot be fed in the water. The above example relates to the penguin pool at Edinburgh Zoo, UK, which has biofiltration and consequently the penguins are hand-fed (Stevenson et al., 1994). This is because penguins often will not consume fish that is not moving. Thus, the way in which we ensure the quality of a substrate can affect the potential to provide behavioural opportunities for captive animals.

Finally, we come to the top substrate or the top of the enclosure. The top substrate could be the highest part of the middle substrate, the sky, an enclosure top, or another type of cover. The top substrate often performs two functions, it restrains the animals movements and it is often the source of light into the enclosure. Light is a very crucial part of any animal enclosure, light permits the animal care-givers to visually inspect the animals (often a requirement under law in many countries) and has a great influence on animal welfare. The characteristics of light that are important are:

- duration of light–dark cycle, this is often linked to the control of behaviour patterns such as reproduction (Cobb et al., 1995; Harvey et al., 1996);
- intensity, how much light the subject receives (Moinard et al., 2001; Davis et al., 1999);
- wavelength composition, light wavelengths can affect the synthesis of vital chemicals in the bodies of some species and may be important in sexual selection, e.g. UV and birds (Maddocks et al., 2001);
- heat, light is often a source of heat within an enclosure (Wheler & Fa, 1995);
- light colour (Lomas et al., 1998);
- presence of dawn and dusk often cue certain types of behaviours such as sleeping or hunting (Lemercier, 2000);
- pattern of light, e.g. solid, random, dappled etc. (Sherwin et al., 1999a).

The characteristics are often overlooked when the lighting regime, if it is even considered, are put into place (Figure 10.1). Often the only concern about light is whether there is sufficient light for humans to observe the animals. In farms, animals housed inside tend to be exposed to low light levels as these often reduce

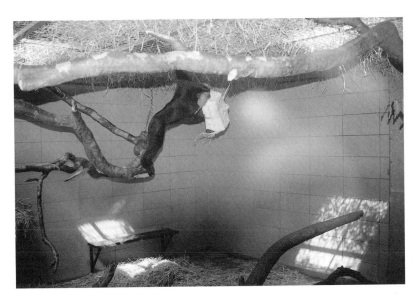

Figure 10.1 Straw on a cage roof is used to lower light levels and provide a dappled effect to mimic forest lighting patterns. The lion-tailed macaque is attempting to get hold of an enrichment feeder (© Robert J. Young).

the level of aggression between group-housed animals (Appleby *et al.*, 1992). In zoos, animals tend to be housed in brightly-lit enclosures surrounded by the public in dimly-lit viewing areas as this facilitates public viewing (Hancocks, 1996). The problem in zoos is perhaps also exacerbated by public perceptions of a species' wild environment, for example, the public expect bats to be housed in darkly lit enclosures but they do not expect forest species such as margays (small exotic cats) to exist in such enclosures. Overall, the main problem seen in zoos is that forest species are often housed in bright enclosures, yet if one visits the rainforest one will discover that it is very dark inside even in the middle of the day with the sun directly overhead. While it is relatively easy to take physical measurements of light in a species' natural environment it is something that is rarely done.

Despite the ease with which light can be measured and the number of studies that demonstrate its importance to a wide range of species characteristics (e.g. health, reproduction, behaviour and welfare; see list above), the only review on the subject I could find was on primates (Erkert, 1989). It seems odd that it has been so ignored by environmental enrichment scientists. There are a few studies that have looked at one or other characteristics of light but none that I know of that have considered it in its totality. For example, one study on chimpanzees showed that their behaviour was much calmer when they were housed under green light (Fritz *et al.*, 1997) but did not consider any other physical characteristics of light. The colour of objects within a enclosure can affect whether animals will use them or not, this usually relates to the animal's ability to camouflage itself on the object (Garrett & Smith, 1994). Light entering an enclosure obviously reflects back from the animal (or is completely absorbed in the case of black species) and species that possess camouflage coats have evolved these under certain light conditions. Thus, enclosures that have the 'wrong' light, principally too bright, may cause a species distress as it perceives itself to be under increased risk of predation (Carlstead *et al.*, 1993).

Some zoos have started to use dappled light for forest species to reduce light levels within enclosures but I know of none that are doing this systematically. Catlow *et al.* (1998) put straw on the wire tops of primate enclosures to create dappled light for forest species. They also report that the straw acted as a substrate onto which food could be thrown, thereby increasing the foraging area for arboreal primates at the appropriate level. Law *et al.* (1997) reported that placing green gardeners' mesh on the top substrate of an enclosure reduced light levels inside (and helped to prevent frost attack on plants). These are a start but the subject of light within animals enclosures deserves further consideration, and a survey of physical light conditions in animal enclosures would be a good starting point for a study. I am positive that in the future greater attention to the physical characteristics of light within a species' enclosure will pay dividends in terms of resolving some health, behaviour and welfare problems (see above). It is already known that UV_B light is important for bone formation of reptiles, especially in species that live close to the equator (Wheler & Fa, 1995). Studies are also revealing a strong link between UV light and how it affects the attractiveness of a bird species to a member of the opposite sex (Bennett *et al.*, 1997): future investigations may reveal the importance of this in the reproduction of captive wild species of birds. Studies on domesticated species of birds have found that UV light is implicated in the development of feather pecking (Sherwin *et al.*, 1999b), an abnormal behavioural pattern that also occurs in exotic pet and zoo housed bird species (van Hoek & King, 1997; Bennett *et al.*, 1997).

Finally, the top substrate may be utilised for arboreally foraging species. Catlow *et al.* (1998) covered the mesh roof of their primate enclosures with straw and onto this straw they scattered the primates' daily food ration. The effect of this roof-top feeding was to allow arboreal primates to feed at a level above the ground. The roof has also been used to locate foraging devices for primates (Brent & Eichberg, 1991). Law has utilised the roof of small-cat enclosures to provide hunting opportunities for small cats by suspending enrichment devices from them (Tudge, 1992). Thus, the roof of an animal's enclosure should not be viewed as useless space.

10.4 Barriers: Keeping People Out and Animals In

The final part of our three-dimensional enclosure is the walls or the surfaces that connect the bottom and top substrates. Often the walls of an enclosure are unutilised space and yet, if an enclosure was a box shape the walls would constitute two thirds of the available surface area. The one primary function of walls, like all terminal substrates, is to keep the animal inside its enclosure. For certain categories and types of animals the walls serve to keep people out and indeed to protect the animals from people; unfortunately, this is especially important for zoo animals (Hediger, 1950; Hediger, 1969; Hediger, 1955). In this context the walls of an enclosure are more properly referred to as barriers. There exists a huge range of barriers, all of which have different properties that can affect animal well-being. The most common types of barriers include:

- metal mesh walls or bars;
- solid walls of brick, plants, metal etc.;
- glass walls, normally reinforced, could be one-way;
- moats, dry or water;
- electric fences;
- piano wire;
- novel barriers.

The type of barrier used is in part dependent upon species' characteristics and upon the use to which humans put that species. Remember, all barriers should permit the human care-giver to view the animals. Principally, large farmed animals are restrained by solid walls or electric fences and small farm animals such as birds by mesh walls. Zoo animals may be restrained by any of the above types of barriers but principally mesh walls, glass walls and moats are used. Laboratory animals are usually constrained by mesh or solid walls. Pets such as domestic cats and dogs may experience no barriers whatsoever but many species are constrained by glass or mesh.

The most common application of barriers that can have things attached to them is to provide climbing surfaces for scansorial species. Edinburgh Zoo, UK has fixed larch poles to the walls of parrot enclosures and ropes to the walls of primate enclosures to promote climbing behaviour (Figure 10.2). Other uses of wall space are possible, for example, a surface onto which visual stimuli can be projected. Barnes and Baron (1961) found that rats seem to derive positive stimulation from looking at the projections of complex objects (for more examples see Anderson, 1998). As always with all environmental enrichment the possibilities are only limited by the human care-givers' imagination.

Mesh and bar walls can be excellent surfaces for scansorial species, although this type of barrier often reminds people of prisons, therefore, organisations such as zoos have shied away from using them. The public's negative associations with bars or mesh is so strong that some zoos have stopped using them completely. Also, with large scansorial species it would also be necessary to use a stand-off barrier (Hancocks, 1996) to prevent human–animal contact. Mesh and bars also provide excellent surfaces for attaching furniture and other forms of envi-

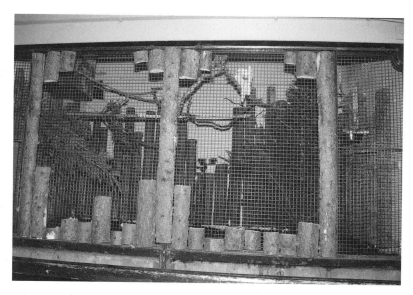

Figure 10.2 Larch pole strips have been attached to the walls of a parrot enclosure to encourage climbing and to increase utilisation of space. (© Robert J. Young).

ronmental enrichment. They also provide animals with the opportunity to view the world outside of their enclosure which, for some species, can be very enriching. Law *et al.*, for example, positioned a tiger enclosure on a hillside to enable the occupants to watch a local horse-riding school adjacent to the zoo (Tudge, 1992), and built a platform that allowed cheetah to watch cars on the nearby motorway (see above and Tudge, 1992). The main problem with bars or mesh is that they do little to prevent the spread of disease. Certain species, primates, for example, are susceptible to human diseases and can potentially pass diseases onto humans.

Normally, solid walls are used with non-scansorial species and the walls are of a sufficient height to keep the animal inside but allow an adult human to see over the top. Thus, in a zoo setting, such types of walls must be used with stand-off barriers to prevent human–animal contact. For laboratory-housed dogs, low walls of this type are excellent for promoting human–animal contact, which can be very important to the dogs' psychological well-being (Loveridge, 1998). These barriers also provide good opportunities for attaching furniture and other forms of enrichment, provided the wall is not covered in a substrate such as ceramic tiles. However, solid walls prevent a species from seeing the world outside its enclosure and for some species, this deprives them of important sensory stimulation (Lyons *et al.*, 1997). These types of walls are better at preventing disease transmission.

Glass walls have often been the favourite of zoos and the public for small pet species, e.g. fish, rodents and reptiles. In these environments people are principally interested in being able to see and potentially interact with animals inside their enclosure. Glass allows people to get very close to animals and provides excellent visual contact without permitting physical contact. Unfortunately, glass barriers seem to encourage people to try and make animals react to their presence, principally by banging on the glass. In studies on fish in a public aquarium, banging on the glass led to increased fish mortality; although signs asking the public not to do so reduced the problem they did not eliminate it (Kratochvil & Schwammer, 1997). The effects of banging on glass walls of other species' enclosures has not been assessed. In some cases zoos have eliminated this problem by erecting stand-off barriers in front of glass walls. Glass barriers obviously provide excellent opportunities for animals to view their outside world and potentially to communicate visually with people (Cook & Hosey, 1995; Hosey, 2000), which may have a negative or positive effect on their welfare. However, glass walls are extremely effective at preventing olfactory and auditory communications (McCune, 1997). In zoos that mainly use glass barriers I often think that visitors must leaving thinking that animals live in a mute world. Thus, the richness of animal communication is often lost to the human observer. This problem can be solved by placing microphones in the animals' enclosures and speakers in the public areas but this is rarely done. Some species of animals, principally reptiles, appear to be unable to perceive the presence of glass as a barrier and may repeatedly rub against it or crash into it causing physical injury (Blake et al., 1998). Usually, glass makes an extremely poor surface for attaching furniture and other forms of enrichment and for most scansorial species it is an unusable substrate or surface. Glass is also perhaps the most labour intensive type of barrier to use as it often requires cleaning several times a day. However, glass can be a good barrier to prevent the spread of disease. It should also be noted that from time to time animal species discover ways of breaking even bomb-proof glass. In some zoos orang-utans, for example, have learnt that a sharp blow with a metal object to the corner of a bomb-proof window will shatter the glass (Markowitz, 1982). Finally, I should comment on the use of one-way glass as it is something that is often discussed by zoos and laboratories for species that are sensitive to human presence, male gorillas, for example. One-way glass works by having the animal in a brightly-lit room and the viewer in a dimly-lit room. From the animal's side the glass appears to be a mirror and from the viewer's side it appears to be a window. (Just think of police movies that feature identity parades.) Immediately, we can see two problems; one, we are placing a species in a brightly lit environment (see above) and two, we are putting a mirror into the species' environment which may cause the species to react to it. Even if these two factors are not a problem for the species concerned, one-way glass is extremely expensive.

The use of moats to restrain the movements of zoo animals was principally started by Carl Hagenbeck when he designed his zoo in Hamburg, Germany (1907) to look like a landscape painting as moats did not disrupt the view of the land-scape (Bostock, 1993). Ever since, moats have been popular with zoos and con-tinue to be so today. There are two basic kind of moats, wet and dry. Obviously, wet moats can only be used for species that do not swim. Both types of moats for reasons of public health and safety, require stand-off barriers. Dry moats tend to be more common because there are fewer problems associated with them. Wet moats can freeze over in the winter, facilitating the escape of animals and in some zoos this is combated by locking the animals inside for the duration of the winter, e.g. the chimpanzee enclosure at a Zoo in the Netherlands (de Waal, 1983), a situation that I believe is not in the best welfare interests of the animals. In a number of zoos animals have fallen into wet moats and drowned. On occasions, social pressures have motivated individual animals to try and cross water moats even though they cannot swim. Water moats also create greater health and safety risks for the public and animal care-givers. However, when integrated properly and well designed they can add significantly to the aesthetics of an enclosure. Some zoos use wet moats as enrichment by throwing floating food onto the surface, chal-lenging the animals to procure the food; however, the risks of drowning should be considered. The first piece of information one requires before constructing a moat is the jumping ability of the species to be contained within the enclosure. In the case of dry moats it is possible to allow the species access to the moat area pro-vided the wall of the moat does not allow the animal to climb out, i.e. the moat is sufficiently deep and its boundary wall smooth. The moat area can provide more space for animals, and potentially an area where they can escape from human or conspecific gaze. Hancock (1996) makes the point that animals such as elephants can be constrained by small moats and suggests that such moats, if not hidden from public view, belittle the power of such animals. Moats do of course provide animals with views of their surroundings and if not too large, the ability to com-municate with other species, including humans, using different sensory modalities (vision, audition and olfaction).

The use of electric fences has become increasing popular with the housing of large outdoor farm and zoo animals (in the UK it is not possible to house labo-ratory animals outdoors) (Chamove, 1998). Electric fences have the beauty of being highly flexible, and it is possible quickly to surround an area with an elec-tric fence to create an enclosure. This can be especially useful for grazing species (e.g. sheep or antelope) or species that can quickly destroy the vegetation in an area (e.g. elephants and goats). Many farmers and zoos use electric fences to rotate animals' use of land. Electric fences have also been employed successfully to restrain the movements of animals such as chimpanzees and wolves. In a zoo envi-ronment an electric fence must be used with a stand-off barrier to prevent the public from receiving shocks. Obviously, electric fences are susceptible to short cir-cuits and other power losses, although systems with back-up power exist and even systems that will phone a number to warn of power failure. The area around an electric fence needs to be kept clear of plants, which can short-circuit the fence. A number of species have learnt how to short-circuit such fences with tools (e.g. the great apes) and some species are, by virtue of their coat, immune to electric shocks, e.g. porcupines whose quills, like the tusks of elephants do not transmit electricity (for further examples see Hancocks, 1996). Thus, the use of an electric fence with a species needs to be carefully considered from an escape and a behavioural point of view. For example, it might be that tool using, such as chimpanzees perform with sticks (Goodall, 1986), is an excellent form of enrichment but one that cannot be used if the barrier is an electric fence. As discussed by Hancocks (1996), electric fences can be almost invisible and therefore aesthetically pleasing. Obviously, one cannot connect anything to them but they do provide for rich sensory communication with the surrounding world (see section on moats above).

Principally for bird species, some zoos have used vertically strung thin wire under high tension to restrain the movements of animals. Again, a stand-off barrier would be necessary in a zoo to prevent human contact. The advantages and disadvantages are similar to those for moats or electric fences but there is perhaps less probability of an animal escape. Aesthetically, the wire can be almost invisible but does require large beams to be fixed to the top and bottom of the enclosure (Hancocks, 1996). The main disadvantage could be that some species will not perceive a barrier to be present and crash into it.

A number of zoos have experimented to varying degrees of success with novel types of barriers. Unfortunately, few of these barriers have been systematically investigated. Apenhaul Zoo in the Netherlands has used behavioural conditioning to keep primates within certain areas of the zoo. Basically, the zoo consists of a series of water-surrounded islands that the public walk through and the animals (only monkey species) live on, the public crossing from one island to another over a metal bridge. The metal bridges can be electrified to condition the animals to stay on their island. Antwerp Zoo experimented with bright lights and found that small birds would stay in brightly lit areas and not fly into dark public areas (Hancocks, 1971). In a laboratory experiment Buchanan-Smith (Buchanan-Smith et al., 1993) found that cotton-top tamarins would avoid the scent of predators. The forestry commission in Scotland has spread lion faeces on trees to prevent damage by red deer, and many zoos do a roaring trade selling lion faeces to gardens as a way of preventing domestic cats entering and using their garden as a latrine. As a consequence, a number of zoos have discussed the use of olfactory barriers based on the use of predator scents from faeces (Epple et al., 1995). To the best of my knowledge, no zoos have put this into practice. Even if such barriers were effective, they could not be supported on animal-welfare grounds as the animals constrained within will be in constant fear of predation thereby breaking one of the Five Freedoms that guard animal welfare. However, such barriers may be useful in keeping free-ranging animals away from certain areas.

Hancocks (1996) has suggested that the ideal barrier would be some kind of force-field but I think he is guilty, as are most architects, of only seeing a barrier from a building and aesthetic perspective. I agree with him wholeheartedly that bars are ugly but the barred gorilla enclosures at Howlett and Port Lympne Zoos, UK, provide far more behavioural opportunities for their occupants than any force-field could. Here, of course, I am conceding the point that environmental education using such exhibits would be difficult (Kreger *et al.*, 1998) but as I have frequently stated, this is a matter of determining priorities for the use to which the animals are being put. Personally, I believe that welfare should always be the number one priority, irrespective of animal use.

10.5 The World Outside the Enclosure

The world surrounding an animal's enclosure is probably as important in having an effect on animal welfare as the enclosure itself (Orgeldinger, 1997; Schapiro *et al.*, 1995; Schapiro *et al.*, 1993). The area around an enclosure could be:

- conspecific animal enclosures;
- contraspecific animal enclosures;
- human care-givers' area;
- public viewing area;
- the natural environment;
- the inside of a room;
- any mixture of the above.

Normally, these areas of the animal's macro-environment have a strong influence on important physical variables in the animals micro-environment (i.e. enclosure) such as temperature, humidity, wind speed etc. However, these areas are also the potential source of a huge amount of sensory stimulation depending on what they contain and the barriers that constrain the animal to its enclosure. Some of this stimulation could be positive for animal welfare and some negative. I will now discuss in turn each of the five types of sensory stimulation potentially emanating from such areas.

Visual stimulation is perhaps the most common since nearly all animal enclosures have the facility for the care-giver to see inside. A number of species appear to react positively to certain kinds of stimulation; for example, chimpanzees will work to open a window that gives them a view of the outside world (Schmitz, 1994). Rats, as already mentioned, appear to be stimulated by looking at complex objects (Barnes & Baron, 1961). However, this does not mean that all visual stimulation is good. Some species of zoo-housed primates become stressed when large, noisy and mobile crowds of people form in front of their enclosure (Wood, 1998; Hosey, 2000; Lambeth *et al.*, 1997; Mitchell *et al.*, 1992; Mitchell *et al.*, 1991; Chamove *et al.*, 1988; Hosey & Druck, 1986). Whereas for other species of mammals, zoo visitors may prove to be a form of environmental enrichment (Hosey, 2000). Many species of animals learn to recognise their veterinarian or care-giver's uniform and

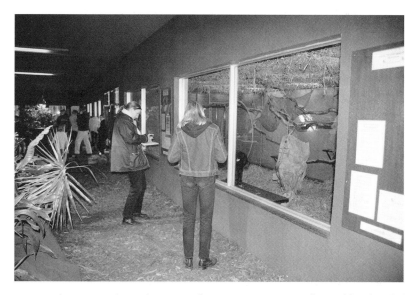

Figure 10.3 Placing people inside a naturalistic viewing area usually modifies their behaviour so that they cause less stress for the animals they are watching. Note the forest bark on the floor, the plants and the low light level (© Robert J. Young).

if this has been associated with negative experiences, such as restraint for medical treatment, can respond to this visual stimulus with fear. Numerous solutions exist to the problems of stress caused by human presence. First, we can minimise the impact of human presence by reducing the time they are in front of an enclosure; some zoos use moving walkways in front of sensitive species' enclosures, such as primates. Second, we can use knowledge from environmental psychology to modify human behaviour so that it disturbs animals minimally. People placed in dark environments that contain things from the natural world usually speak quietly and behave in a calm manner (Maple & Findlay, 1989; see Figure 10.3). Third, we can habituate animals to care-giver or veterinarian's uniforms.

A second important source of visual stimulation is other animal species. How this stimulation is perceived depends on the relationships between the species but possibilities are: predator and prey, conspecific competitor, contraspecific competitor, neutral, dominant and subordinate. This again is an area that has not been systematically studied by scientists so I can only make some suggestions that need to be investigated. Law *et al.* (1997) have suggested that it is stimulating for large carnivores to see prey species and has designed enclosures to afford such opportunities. Others have considered this frustrating for the carnivore and stressful for the prey species. Further studies are clearly needed to resolve these arguments as presently we only have indirect or non-empirical evidence. Mason (1991) in her review of stereotypic animal behaviour found many examples that were apparently induced by frustration. However, Law (personal communication) never saw his tigers performing any abnormal behaviour but did not systematically observe them. In the zoo and laboratory communities it is widely recognised that visual contact between competitors or dominants and subordinates causes stress (Crockett, 1998). It is for this reason that these organisations generally erect visual barriers between such animals, the most common case being between large carnivores, who are often observed to pace along an area from where they can see another large carnivore species (Veasey, 1993). An interesting exception to this case is the territorial behaviour of some species. Edinburgh Zoo deliberately housed two Diana monkey groups in visual contact to promote territorial behaviour, the rationale being that it would promote important social behaviour, i.e. the group territorial protection displays of females, and thereby enhance group unity. (Unfortunately, this situation was not systematically investigated.) In this case, both groups could easily move out of visual contact with the other group if they so desired. Blake *et al.* (1998) have argued that in mixed-species exhibits of reptiles, the movements of one species may provide positive stimulation for another. A number of studies on domestic horses solitary-housed in boxes report reduced incidence of behavioural problems (e.g. stereotypies) when the horses can see conspecifics (Winskill *et al.*, 1995). Cooper *et al.* (2000) found that even just the ability to view the outside world had an effect on reducing stereotypic behaviour in solitary-housed horses. Before I finish this section on visual stimulation, I would like to remind the reader that the visual perception of different species is very different from humans, some are colour blind, others have black and white vision, some have greater visual acuity, others less. Finally, if we are aware of the importance of visual stimulation then we have the possibility of designing environments that are positively stimulating (i.e. enriching).

Animal species often receive unintentional and sometimes intentional auditory stimuli from their macro-environment (Schaffer *et al.*, 2001; Sales *et al.*, 1999; Milligan *et al.*, 1993). Again, it is worth pointing out that many animal species have the ability to hear frequencies above and below that which human hearing can perceive. Just as certain frequencies and volume of sound can be distressing to humans, the same is true of animal species. It is well established that certain frequencies of ultrasound can cause severe distress to rodent species. The most well known example being the unintentional production of ultrasound when water is running from a tap. If a chipmunk is housed in a room with a television left in standby mode, the ultrasound produced by the television can kill the animal within two days (Meredith, 2002). Unfortunately, there are many potential anthropogenic sound sources in an animal's environment: the sound of equipment, vehicles and radios. Not only can the frequencies of anthropogenic sounds cause stress but they can also disrupt vocal communication between animals and this may have negative effects on animal welfare. In one study, the noise from fans in a farrowing house was shown to interfere in sow and piglet vocal communication during suckling (Algers & Jensen, 1991).

It is often best to discourage the use of radios by animal care-givers unless they have been shown to have beneficial effects for that species (see below; Newberry, 1995; Lemercier, 2000). In terms of machinery and vehicles, it should be possible to use soundproofing to minimise their effects. It is not only possible that machines and vehicles produce stressful sound frequencies but also sounds that initiate animal vocalisations. Diesel tractors can initiate the territorial vocalisation of masked titi monkeys, a species that rarely comes into visual contact with conspecifics. (Interestingly, this species has proved very difficult to keep alive let alone breed in captivity.) Field scientists have often reported that the 'turning-over' of their car engine can initiate territorial calling in howler monkey, a species that does relatively well in captivity. Thus, the adverse properties of sound on animal well-being should never be underestimated.

In an unpublished study, there is an example of anthropogenic sound, music, having a positive effect on animals. It has been reported that playing slow music (less than 100 beats per minute) to cattle increased their milk yield (Adrian North, University of Leicester, UK, 2001). A number of zoos have experimented with playing music or naturalistic sounds to animals as a form of enrichment with varying degrees of success, often reporting more calm behaviour in the animals (Ogden *et al.*, 1994). A number of laboratories that house primates in groups have found that playing human voices, on a random schedule, to primates in the absence of human care-givers reduces aggression (personal observation). This effect appears to be due to the fact that the animals have learnt that human care-givers will stop fights.

Sound pollution from other animal species, including conspecifics, can also occur. Depending on the relationship between the species, the effects of these calls can be positive, negative or neutral (irrelevant). If the animal calls have a positive effect then we can use playback of these calls to enrich the animal's life. The most commonly used example is the playback of territorial songs to gibbon species (Maples *et al.*, 1988). However, we need to be careful that we playback at ambient volumes so as not to cause stress – the volume of a call can relate to the size of the caller. It is also important not to use playback too often or the animals will habituate to it. Thus, an abnormally loud territorial call could make the target animal perceive that there is an enormous competitor nearby. Some animals can count the number of animals calling (McComb *et al.*, 1994), and if this is greater than their group size this could be threatening to them. The infrequent use of predator calls can be useful in stimulating vigilance in captive animals. Chamove and Moodie (1990) have argued that short-duration threatening events can be stimulating and enriching to captive animals.

Some animal-rights groups have suggested that animal enclosures, a pool for a killer whale, for example, cause welfare problems due to sound echoing back from hard surfaces. However, I know of no scientific studies that have investigated this possibility. We do, however, know that restrictive environments can modify not only the context of animal vocalisations but also their frequency. This has been suggested to have adverse consequences on the ability of such species to survive reintroduction (Castro *et al.*, 1998). It is well established in the scientific literature that the frequencies that animals use when vocalising have been selected by evolution to ensure maximum propagation in the species' wild habitat. Thus, animal vocalisations are said to utilise sound windows that differ between open, e.g. savannah, and closed habitats, e.g. forests (Waser & Brown, 1984).

Olfactory stimuli are very important for many animal species as such stimuli can provide a wealth of information about resources such as food and the presence of conspecifics. Many species of animal primarily use their sense of smell to detect food; it is easy to identify such species as they usually have a pronounced snout with a wet nose. Obviously, this should suggest to us important methods of enriching their environments, e.g. food trails for hunting carnivores. It should also make us aware of potential welfare problems (Sommerville & Broom, 1998); for example, some species of farm animals (e.g. breeding sows and broiler breeders) are heavily food restricted for reasons of fertility and economics (Young, 1999). Other species, such as bears, are hyperphagic (i.e. have a constant hunger) due to their life-history strategy of hibernating during the winter months when food is unavailable. In both of these cases, therefore, it is important to consider the position of food stores in relation to animal enclosures and prevailing local wind direction. It has been suggested to me by bear keepers that stereotypic route pacing by bears is caused by the frustration of smelling inaccessible food. However, this hypothesis needs to be tested.

Many species use olfaction to communicate important information about themselves, such as their territorial area, their social status, their reproductive status etc. In the case of environmental marking by animals, such signals might work over only a short distance but in the case of pheromones they can work over a long distance. Perhaps one of the most important olfactory signals a species emits is its territorial marking as this serves to keep competitors away. It is important, therefore, that when we clean animal enclosures we are not constantly removing their territorial scents as this is likely to be stressful. It has been suggested that in cages for (laboratory) mice only half the area of the cage at any one point in time should be cleaned (van Loo *et al.*, 2000; Saibaba *et al.*, 1996; Nevison *et al.*, 1999). Whether or not we promote other types of olfactory social signals depends on our objectives for particular animals. If, for example, we wish to pair asocial species for breeding then such olfactory communication would be vital. However, if we did not wish to breed such species then the transmission of such olfactory signals could be very frustrating for the animals. This type of frustration could induce abnormal behaviour (Mason, 1991). Clearly, we need to think a great deal about olfactory communication when we are designing animal environments. The final source of olfactory stimulation I wish to mention is that produced by substrates and plants within a species enclosure. For example, catnip (*Nepeta cataria*) is known to induce play or kitten like behaviour in felid species. Law and Tatner (1998) have suggested this can be used to help introduce large, potentially aggressive felids (such as clouded leopards) to each other for breeding. It is worth mentioning at this point that the response of felids to catnip is dependent on the possession of a particular gene (Law *et al.*, 1998). Not all such olfactory sources are positive for welfare (see above) and can disrupt the olfactory field of a species.

The final two senses, touch and taste, are perhaps the least understood of all in terms of their implications for animal welfare. Taste is perhaps best dealt with in the section concerning feeding enrichment (see Chapter 8). The sense of touch is perhaps most often stimulated by the substrates in the species enclosure. Only one study has directly examined tactile qualities in environmental enrichment (Rice *et al.*, 1999). However, a number of scientists have experimented with the choice tests to determine which substrates species such as battery hens (Hughes & Duncan, 1988), domestic horses (Mills *et al.*, 2000), or domestic cats (Hawthorne *et al.*, 1997) most prefer. These tests tell us which of a given range of choices the animal finds least aversive but they tell us nothing about their relative sensory properties to animals. Also, it is possible that the substrates that animals prefer are not the best for their physical well-being. Bumble-foot, a disease of captive birds, is thought to result from under-use of the foot or stimulation of circulation in the foot. In species such as penguins the probability of the disease developing can be reduced by using a stone-covered substrate for the animals to walk on but the animals may prefer to walk on a substrate such as smooth concrete. It is worth mentioning at this point that the different materials from which we construct a species enclosure have different physical properties that can affect animal welfare (Heidbrink, 1997). Here I am not only thinking about texture but also about other relevant properties such as thermal properties (e.g. heat retention) and ease of cleaning (e.g. waterproofing and durability). Some species use their sense of touch to navigate in their environment, e.g. snakes (Chiszar *et al.*, 1987), or to find resources, e.g. ayes-ayes to find food (Sterling & Povinelli, 1999). Obviously we need to consider such behavioural predispositions when designing a species' enclosure.

10.6 Conclusion

This chapter, I hope, will stimulate and guide people in designing enriched environments for the species in their care. While I have not given species-specific guidance due to the scale of the problem (i.e. 10000 species of birds, 4000 species of mammals etc.) I hope the contents of this chapter will guide and stimulate the reader to think in a systematic and objective manner about animal environments.

Furniture, Toys and other Objects

In Chapter 10 I considered the substrates, the levels that make up the animal's enclosure and some of the permanent physical features that make up an animal's enclosure. In Portuguese, the word for furniture is 'móveis', which literally translates to movable things; the word for flats or houses is 'imóveis', non-movable things. I will discuss below situations which demonstrate that the static nature of animal enclosures need not be so. In this chapter I wish to focus on the things that we can put inside, take away and change within an animal's enclosure – its furniture.

11.1 Furniture

The furniture within an enclosure is important in improving the quality of space and consequently, the quality of life that the occupants experience. The provision of furniture within a species' enclosures should be both species-specific and goal-specific. For example, the furniture for giant panda in a zoo should reflect the species' requirements (e.g. to forage for bamboo) and the reasons for their captivity (e.g. captive breeding, research or environmental education). Given this information we can decide what furniture this species requires when housed for this goal. In Table 11.1 I have listed the main behaviour patterns that furniture can be used to facilitate the expression of or to stimulate. It should of course be noted that furniture is not necessary to stimulate every behaviour pattern of every species. For example, lions only require an appropriate substrate on which to lie to facilitate sleep.

Ideally, animals would be provided with all their furniture requirements but for economic, practical and other reasons this is not always possible. In terms of prioritising the furniture an animal requires we can use their hierarchy of needs: physiological (life-sustaining), safety (health-sustaining) and behavioural (comfort-sustaining; Table 11.2 & Figures 11.1–11.2).

Table 11.1 Furniture used to facilitate behaviour expression.

Behaviour	Example Furniture
Avoiding predators	Vegetation, climbing frames, perches, hide boxes, visual barriers
Birthing	Dens, nest boxes, plants
Cognition	Puzzle feeders
Comfort	Scratching posts, showers, wallows
Drinking	Ponds, water moats, nipple drinkers
Eliminative	Litter trays
Exploration	Toys, novel objects
Finding food	Foraging devices, foraging boards, feeders, bowls, plants
Learning	Puzzle feeders, toys, novel objects
Locomotion	Climbing frames, perches, vegetation, hunting enrichment, foraging enrichment, swimming pools
Marking	Wooden posts, plants, general furniture
Play	Toys, novel objects, plants
Shelter	Nest boxes, dens, man-made shelters, plants, grottos, tunnels
Sleep	Platforms, shelves, nest boxes, beds
Social avoidance	Hide boxes, climbing frames, visual barriers
Social interaction	Resting platforms, climbing frames, toys, novel objects, puzzle feeders, grooming boards
Thermal regulation	Shelters, hot rocks
Vigilance	Platforms, plants, climbing frames

Table 11.2 A hierarchy for prioritising furniture requirements of animals (after Duncan & Fraser, 1997).

Physiological or Life-sustaining furniture	Safety or Health-sustaining furniture	Behavioural or Comfort-sustaining furniture
Feeders	Hide boxes	Scratching posts
Drinkers	Nest boxes or dens	Puzzle feeders (to provide
Shelter	Resting areas e.g. platforms	cognitive stimulation)
Sources of warmth	Visual barriers	Toys (for play and exploration)
	Climbing structures	Sensory stimulation
	Opportunity to exercise body	Novel objects (for exploration)
	Scent-marking posts	

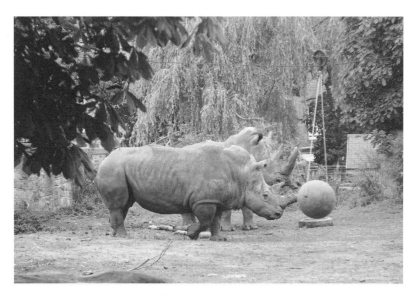

Figure 11.1   Rhinos appear to enjoy hitting large objects with their horn; here the ball is attached to a wire for safety reasons (photograph courtesy of P. Gordon McLeod ©).

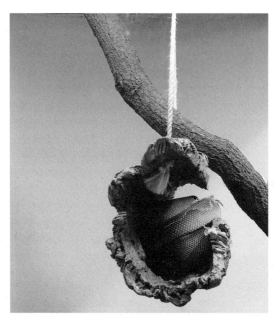

Figure 11.2   A snake resting inside a den after it has made use of the climbing structure in the background (photograph courtesy of P. Gordon McLeod ©).

A key characteristic of furniture is that it is moveable enabling the position of furniture to be altered within an enclosure to provide a source of environmental enrichment. The position of food, water or furniture associated with thermoregulation can be moved within the enclosure to promote exploratory behaviour, for example. The actual physical structure or other physical characteristics of furniture can be varied, the climbing structure provided to primates, for example. Primates that evolved to live in forest environments need to learn routes through the trees and learn when such routes change, e.g. due to broken branches. Thus, these species are constantly updating their spatial map of the environment. The provision of an unvarying climbing frame, no matter how complex, will eventually cease to challenge the cognitive mapping abilities of primates. Therefore, the construction of a climbing frame that can be altered will provide a constant opportunity to stimulate such cognitive challenges. For example, by constructing a climbing frame of wooden branches that are connected together using chains rather than fixed metal posts (Catlow, 1997). Furniture such as toys can also be added to or taken away from the enclosure to provide a source of enrichment (see below).

11.2 Furniture Design and Behaviour

The design of furniture should follow the advice I gave in Chapter 5 for the design of environmental enrichment devices, i.e. it should be goal-driven and concerned about safety issues. The behaviour of furniture when it is utilised by an animal must reflect the function of the furniture and the thing that it is replacing from the species' wild environment. A climbing frame within a primate enclosure is replacing trees. What are the important behavioural characteristics of such structures? Trees are made up of a trunk, branches, twigs and leaves. The trunk is usually of a large diameter, pointing primarily in a vertical direction (90 degrees from the ground) and usually does not move in response to the weight of primates climbing on it. Usually, the trunk of a tree terminates above the ground in a formation of large diameter branches (or boughs) that point upwards at various angles between the near vertical and horizontal and such branches usually do not move under the weight of the primate. Further along these large branches smaller diameter branches emerge at angles also varying from near vertical to horizontal, these branches often move in response to the primate's weight. This pattern of smaller branches emerging from larger ones may be repeated several times until we have reached the twigs and leaves. The smaller the diameter of the branch or the greater the weight of the primate, the greater the movement that can be generated in the branch. Also, the further the primate moves along a small diameter branch the more the branch will move. In many species of trees the high density of branches means that when one branch moves other branches close to this branch will also move. The leaves that obviously move in response to a climbing primate, provide cover from the sun, predators and other conspecifics as well as being food for some species.

In the above description we have captured the functionality (important features) of a climbing structure for primates by describing a tree from a climbing primate's perspective. To summarise, the key characteristics of a primate climbing frame are:

(1) different diameters of the climbing structures;
(2) different angles of climbing structures;
(3) the change in characteristics 1 and 2 as height increases;
(4) the increase in movement of climbing structures as their diameter decreases;
(5) the increased movement of climbing structures as one moves to the detached end;
(6) the possibility that climbing on one branch will cause other branches to move;
(7) access to spatially complex structures with multiple routes;
(8) the provision of cover.

Do these features of a tree really need to be built into a climbing frame? I will answer this question by looking at each feature in turn.

(1) Different diameters affect the way in which the primate can climb, on a wide trunk it may use all four limbs, whereas on a thicker branch it may brachiate. Thus, this feature promotes different forms of natural locomotive behaviour.
(2) Different angles of branches require the primate to use different amounts of energy when climbing and different angles may be associated with different locomotive behaviour. Thus, this feature promotes greater levels of exercise and a variety of natural locomotive behaviours.
(3) The change in branch angles and diameters as a tree grows means that primates must learn these relationships to move successfully in trees. Thus, this feature promotes learning behaviour.
(4) Thinner branches move more than thicker branches, requiring greater balance and strength from the primate. The movement of branches, therefore, promotes strength and hand–eye coordination.
(5) Branches move more as a primate moves along them and are more likely to break. Thus, primates learn about the physical characteristics of their world and increase their level of exercise when climbing on such branches.
(6) Branches can be caused to move when another primate is climbing nearby. Thus, primates learn to be alert to the behaviour of individuals close to them in a tree.
(7) A tree may have thousands of possible routes between two different points due to the large number of branches, i.e. trees are often spatially complex structures. Thus, this feature challenges the primates' spatial learning and spatial memory.
(8) Leaves, if present, can provide the primate with protection from a stressful event. Thus, the absence of cover may make a climbing structure undesirable.

In the example above I have only considered a tree from the point of view of locomotion. In terms of another behaviour pattern, such as nesting, I would need to describe a whole new set of characteristics, such as the ability of branches to be folded. Obviously, if we are really serious about providing furniture for animals we use the natural structure wherever possible since the complexity of creating artificial structures can be enormous, as illustrated by the example above. However, when the natural solution cannot be used we need to view the furniture replacement from the animal's perspective. In laboratory environments, it is not necessary to make an artificial climbing structure look like a tree as laboratories are not trying to convey messages about conservation to the public (Kreger *et al.*, 1998). Some zoos have created artificial trees (I still find it difficult to understand why) from a variety of materials including fibreglass. In one case an expensive full-scale fibreglass tree was placed into an orang-utan's enclosure only for the zoo to discover that fibreglass was too slippery for the orang-utan to grasp. We need to consider carefully, therefore, the materials that furniture is made from (see Chapter 5).

Analysis of furniture from the animal's perspective also reveals the complex and interacting benefits that an animal can receive from climbing something as apparently simple as a tree. In our example above the benefits were: promoting a range of different locomotive behaviours, increase in physical strength, increase in hand–eye coordination, stimulation of cognitive and memory abilities (especially spatial), increased sense of security (see Chapter 3). All too often climbing frames are rigid metal structures formed into a series of cubes and made of uniform pieces of metal. The only benefit of this type of structure is a limited ability to increase the physical strength of primates. Tudge (1992) notes that primates reared on such metal structures find it difficult to climb and navigate within trees and for primates destined for reintroduction this may be a serious problem.

The design and behaviour of furniture is critical in determining its success as environmental enrichment. The exact properties of a piece of furniture that make it a useful piece of environmental enrichment are often complex and require an animal's perspective on the world. Wherever possible we should strive to use Nature's furniture store as this is a far simpler and cheaper solution to the provision of furniture. It should be noted, however, that for animals not all trees are equal. For example, I have seen collared anteaters (an arboreal species) in zoos provided with trees whose bark is too smooth for them to obtain a grip in order to climb.

11.3 Toys and Novel Objects

In this section I am going to equate toys with being novel objects since they share many of the same properties when first introduced into animal enclosures. Initially, animals unaccustomed to toys or novel objects may show an avoidance response that decreases over a period of hours or days (Shimoji *et al.*, 1993). This may be followed by tentative exploration of the toy or object before it is used. Animals accustomed to toys or novel objects may respond by immediately exploring the object (or engaging in object play, see below) or displaying signs of excitement, such as locomotor play (see below; Wood-Gush & Vestergaard, 1991; Wood-Gush & Vestergaard, 1993). The obvious difference between toys and novel objects is that animals learn and remember what the toy does, i.e. which behaviour pattern it stimulates, and how the toy functions. Thus, along with exploration and signs of excitement, toys should also generate the expression of specific behaviour patterns (see below); they will have some ability to reduce general levels of fear but not as greatly as novel objects (since they are only novel on first presentation). Thus, in the programme of toy implementation I outline below, one could consider on certain days using a novel object instead of a toy but it may prove difficult to keep finding novel objects to utilise.

The addition of toys to an animal's environment is perhaps the most commonly employed form of environmental enrichment. This application of toys no doubt reflects their widespread availability, simplicity of use (just put it in the enclosure) and familiarity to us from human society. In general, we tend to think of toys as objects that stimulate play behaviour (Hubrecht, 1993; Garner *et al.*, 1996). Play can be divided into three main types: solitary locomotor play (e.g. the gambolling of dairy calves); object play (which may be social, e.g. tug-of-war games between dogs, or non-social, e.g. the chasing of a ball of wool by cats); social, e.g. chase games between chimpanzees (Fagen, 1992). In this section we are primarily interested in object play since we are discussing the value of toys to animal welfare.

Why do animals play? It should be pointed out that current knowledge suggests that only mammals and birds play but Burghardt *et al.* (1996) have suggested that reptiles also play but this opinion is not widely accepted. One of the main reasons for animal play is that it provides the animal with the opportunity to practice the behavioural skills that it needs for survival (Harcourt, 1991; Spijkerman *et al.*, 1996; Spinka *et al.*, 2001). Object play principally involves the manipulation of the objects, which helps to develop locomotor and visual system coordination. If we look in detail at object play we can often recognise the underlying behaviour pattern that the animal is practising. In carnivores, object play often resembles the hunting behaviour of the species concerned. Domestic cats strike, chase and pounce on balls of wool. Polar bears take hold of large balls in their pool and shake them vigorously up and down in the water, which is one method they use for killing seals, literally shaking the air out of them (Stirling, 1990). Dogs, primates and other species often use objects as the focus of social interactions, such as tug-of-war or chase games. The expression of such games may facilitate the development of social skills, social knowledge and help in the formation of social hierarchies. Chase games may also help in the development of anti-predator behaviour.

The problem with object play is differentiating it from simple object interaction. Most animal species, even fish and insects, will interact with objects in their environment usually by attempting to move them (this is what Burghardt *et al.*, 1996 reported as play in reptiles) but this is not play. High levels of object play are usually only seen in species with advanced cognitive abilities, such as primates, cetaceans and elephants (Lewis, 2000). However, the amount of time an animal spends utilising an enrichment technique does not necessarily reflect the importance of that technique for animal welfare. Thus, all mammal and bird species can benefit from the effects of toys. It should also be pointed out that play behaviour is much more common in juvenile animals than it is in adults; in some species adults may only show play behaviour when interacting with juveniles. Thus, the value of play to animals appears to vary with age (Spinka *et al.*, 2001; Smith *et al.*, 1996; Markus & Croft, 1995). Notable exceptions to this rule are some domesticated pet species, especially dogs and cats, which appear to have been selected for high levels of play in adulthood. Play is seen as highly desirable behaviour in pets, especially if humans can engage the species in play (Rooney & Bradshaw, 2002; Rooney *et al.*, 2000).

Does the expression of play behaviour have any relationship to animal welfare? A number of scientists have sought to determine whether the occurrence of play can be used as an animal-welfare indicator (see Chapter 3; Fraser & Duncan, 1998). None of these studies have been conclusive. The expression of play seems to be primarily influenced by: the rearing history of the animals (those from barren environments engage in less play); the nutritional energy available to the animals (low food availability usually equates to less play); the opportunity to engage in play, i.e. an environment that has space for locomotor activity, objects that can act as toys and social companions (Jensen & Kyhn, 2000; Jensen *et al.*, 1998; Schapiro *et al.*, 1996; Markus & Croft, 1995; Barrett *et al.*, 1992). However, play can be deemed a 'desirable' behaviour in accordance with the criteria established by Chamove and Anderson (1989), from this perspective we can regard the expression of play as an animal-welfare indicator (see Chapter 3). Furthermore, it could be argued that the provision of toys provides animals with the opportunity to interact with, and express some control over their environment. In Chapter 3, we discussed how control over the environment is one of the main ways that environmental enrichment improves animal welfare.

Since play behaviour is the practising of a variety of behavioural skills (Spinka *et al.*, 2001), we should think about the use of different toy types to promote the expression of different behaviour patterns and not simply provide the animal with a series of random objects. I have already mentioned that much object play behaviour relates to the development of food acquiring or food manipulation skills but this does not mean that play objects need to dispense food (see Chapter 5). Object play can also be related to the development of social skills (see examples above). Toys can also have an effect in developing the expression of exploratory behaviour and the gathering of environmental information (Wemelsfelder & Birke,

1997). Thus, we need to think about toys as objects to elicit particular patterns of play behaviour.

One well known characteristic of toys is that over relatively short periods of time, often less than one day, they are no longer used by the animals or human children for that matter (Crockett, 1998; Wemelsfelder & Birke, 1997). In the case of human children we suggest that this is because they are bored of that toy. Why toys become less attractive to animals is less clear; whether animals can experience the state of boredom is a highly controversial subject and one that we may never be able to answer (but see Wemelsfelder, 1997). It may be that toys are only a source of secondary reinforcement, i.e. reinforcement associated with a primary reinforcer such as food (see Chapter 5; Chance, 1998) and this low level of reinforcement is not enough to maintain high levels of use. In the wild, the successful hunting behaviour of a cat would be reinforced by the consumption of food. Motivational studies with farmed mink demonstrate that toys are not a highly valued resource by this species (Cooper & Mason, 2000). Thus, toys are classified by mink as 'luxury' items (see Chapter 4), which for animals that have an excess of 'free time', means that they are important in improving the welfare status of such a species (Hughes & Duncan, 1988).

Animal-keeping institutions and pet owners usually make the same mistake when implementing toys in their animals' environment. Many different types of toys are normally given to the animals at the same time and then the toys are left in the enclosure for weeks, months or even years. The result of this is that the toys eventually 'migrate' to the corner of the enclosure and are not used again by the animals; in some cases the animal care-giver may remove the 'unwanted' toys. I have already mentioned that toys have a limited period of time that they are attractive to animals, typically less than one day. The effectiveness of toys can be increased by placing only a few toys that are designed to elicit particular behaviour patterns each day and then at the end of the day or the next day removing these toys. The next day different types of toys should be added to the enclosure, and again removed after a maximum of 24 hours. This process should continue to be repeated for at least two weeks before the same toys are once again placed within the animal's enclosure. To achieve the programme outlined one obviously needs a large number of toys. However, the number of toys needed can be reduced by not employing toys as environmental enrichment every day and occasionally using a novel object.

The programme I have outlined for the management of toys obviously will result in a continuous level of change, which if managed incorrectly could be a source of stress (Crockett, 1998). Animals may show fear of such toys in the same way that novel objects can arouse fear. Shimoji *et al.* (1993) report a case of a macaque showing fear reactions to a perch but this was because the animal had always lived in an unchanging environment. It has been shown that repeated exposure of animals to toys (which to the animal are initially novel objects) reduces the animals' future fear of novel objects (Jones & Waddington, 1992) and the animals may show signs of 'excitement' when they see a novel object (Wood-Gush & Vestergaard, 1991; Wood-Gush & Vestergaard, 1993). Furthermore, once a toy is no longer novel it is highly likely that the animals remember both its appearance and function. (In my experience working with a wide variety of animals, they appear to remember how to use a puzzle feeder, for example, immediately upon presentation even if they have had no exposure to it for a year.) The implementation of toys should follow the procedure for implementing new enrichment objects that I outlined in Chapter 6. Thus, the implementation of toys needs managing to ensure their effectiveness as environmental enrichment.

11.4 Alternatives to Static Homes

The concept of an animal's enclosure seems to rely much on our own concept of a home. The enclosure is divided usually into two parts, an inside and an outside area, the inside area often being subdivided into different areas for different functions, e.g. a sleeping box. This concept is rather static and there is no reason why an enclosure should be totally immobile. The simplest method that has been used to vary the enclosure of animals is to rotate them between adjacent enclosures. This is something practised in a number of zoos but not something that I am aware has been systematically investigated. The idea being to provide not only new surroundings to the animal but new sensory experiences (Mellen *et al.*, 1998). Many species leave sensory information in their enclosures which, if not removed by cleaning, could prove to be highly stimulating for the next occupant. Imagine the stimulation a fossa (a cat-like Madagascan carnivore) would receive from exploring an enclosure recently occupied by lemurs (its prey and a species which performs much scent marking (Richards, 1985)). Of course, the transference of species between enclosures must be done in such a way that the new occupant is not exposed to any health risks from the old occupants, e.g. the transmission of parasites. The nature of the stimulation provided should be given careful consideration; lemurs moved into a fossa enclosure may become highly stressed (see Buchanan-Smith *et al.*, 1993, for an example of analogous situation). A territorial cat species moved into a conspecific's enclosure may also become stressed upon smelling fresh scent marks (McCune, 1997) which act as territorial markers. As a general rule, we can move predator species to prey-species enclosures, and rotate species or conspecifics who normally do not have negative interactions, e.g. highly sociable and non-territorial. The actual moving of a species to a new enclosure can cause acute stress, therefore, the frequency of moving animals between enclosures should not be too high (Crockett, 1998), probably a maximum of four times per year. Obviously, animals should not be moved to new enclosures when they are conducting seasonal courtship behaviour (e.g. parrots) or when they have dependent offspring which they are denning (e.g. cats).

One interesting solution to the static home problem that has been used by zoos and laboratories is to connect a series of animal enclosures together. The National Zoo in Washington, DC (USA) has a series of physically separated orang-utan enclosures that are connected by ropes suspended many metres above the ground. The orang-utans can move between the enclosures by swinging along the ropes. The height of the ropes above the ground is such that the orang-utans will not deliberately drop to the ground and the ropes actually pass over the public areas. Thus, the orang-utans have the possibility of changing enclosures and having social encounters with only those individuals that they desire, i.e. it provides the animals with control over social encounters which is very important for animal welfare (see Chapter 3). Laboratories have been able to set up a similar situation by connecting a series of enclosures using ventilation ducting, e.g. the cotton-top tamarin colony that was housed in the University of Stirling, UK (Price & McGrew, 1990). There exists modular rodent housing that allows the owner to buy and connect together by plastic tunnels different enclosures. I believe this concept of multiple-connected enclosures has much promise in terms of improving animal welfare since it gives choice and control back to the animals. Each connected enclosure for group housed animals should contain the basic requirements for survival, i.e. food, water and shelter, to facilitate choice concerning social companionship but this is obviously not important for solitary-housed species. The approach of using interconnected enclosures may be especially useful in zoos or laboratories with limited space that wish to expand the space allowance of a particular species.

A number of laboratories and a few zoos have created playrooms for animals, usually primates, cats and dogs (Holst, 1997; Brent, 1997). These are rooms with high levels of enrichment devices and other sorts of environmental stimulation to which the animals are given access for short periods of time. This can be a highly effective way of providing environmental enrichment when space is highly limited. Obviously, such playrooms can provide access to enrichment to much larger numbers of animals than could be achieved by putting the enrichment into the animals' home enclosures. Thus, for laboratories especially, this solution is highly cost-effective and it is perhaps something which the agricultural industry could consider implementing. Another solution to limited space problems that has been used by a number of zoos is the time-sharing of enclosures (Mellen et al., 1998). At a Zoo in the UK, gorillas and bonobos share the same outside enclosure. It would obviously be better if both parties had their own outside enclosure that they could time-share during the period of a day. However, it may be that the evidence of the other species is stimulating to the species that is currently occupying the outside enclosure. Mellen et al. (1998) reported that a male and female tiger time-sharing the same enclosure took great interest in the scent markers left by the other individual.

There is also the possibility with some species for eliminating completely the use of an enclosure and instead provisioning the animals with food and shelter to make them stay within certain geographical limits, i.e. free-ranging (Beresford-

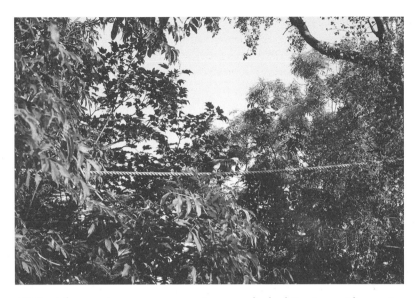

Figure 11.3 A free-ranging cotton-top tamarin; one radical solution to providing environmental enrichment is to dispense with the animal's enclosure completely (© Robert J. Young).

Stoke, 1994; Stafford *et al.*, 1994; Figure 11.3). The camel-herding people of north Africa have used such a system for centuries, but the camels find their own food. It has most commonly been implemented in zoos with small primate species (e.g. tamarins), small deer species (e.g. hog deer), small rodents (e.g. agoutis), flightless birds (e.g. rheas) and even flying bird species (e.g. American night herons). These animals gain the benefits of Nature's furniture store, variability and environmental complexity, all of which should improve animal welfare. However, they are also potentially exposed to the less animal-welfare-friendly aspect of the wild environment: disease, parasitism, predators, thermal discomfort and hunger. Beresford-Stoke (1994) reviewing literature on the free-ranging of primates, found a number of cases where individuals had disappeared, been preyed upon, become ill, become trapped in a predator's enclosure and suffered physical injuries as a result of free-ranging. Thus, the free-ranging of animals needs careful management to ensure that they are not suffering, it should certainly not be viewed as a panacea to animal-welfare problems or as an easy alternative to enclosure housing.

11.5 Conclusion

The static concept of animal housing both in terms of the physical structure and the furniture probably resulted from the ease of management this situation presents, the minimising of labour costs (see Chapter 7) and in my opinion, the erroneous belief that predictable environments are better for animal welfare (Wiepkema, 1990; Young, 1993; Chapter 3) which in practice has been translated into unchanging environments. It is undeniable that too much change, and change over which the animals have no control, can seriously impair animal welfare (Crockett, 1998). However, the implications of this are that we manage change in animal environments and do not create static environments.

Designing and Analysing Enrichment Studies

12

The design and statistical analyses of environmental enrichment studies seem to be the area that causes the greatest fear in people working in this subject area, perhaps because it involves some mathematics. However, given the widespread availability of statistical software and data-processing programmes, such fear is unfounded. Using statistics is now rather like driving a car, you need to know where the controls are and what each control does but not necessarily the fine details of how they operate. It is now the same with statistics, you need to know which test to use and what it basically does, but you do not necessarily need to understand the underlying mathematical equations. (Certainly you should never need to do the calculations of such equations, although personally, I have found this gives me a greater understanding of the statistical tests.) In this chapter I provide a basic model for the reader to follow if they wish to conduct and analyse environmental enrichment studies. It is my hope that by using this model the reader will gain confidence and develop their knowledge way beyond what I have presented here.

12.1 Experimental Design

The scientific validation of environmental enrichment, and various ways it is employed, is of great importance if we are concerned with making real improvements in animal welfare. Some institutions will permit only scientifically validated methods of environmental enrichment to be applied, an approach to be applauded provided such institutions are active in their implementation of environmental enrichment. The problem we face is that it is easier and considerably quicker to think up and devise new forms of environmental enrichment than it is assess their animal-welfare impact. Here we are faced with a dilemma: do we, (a) wait until a new environmental enrichment idea can be systematically and empirically tested before implementing it, or (b) take a chance and implement it without scientific testing. The answer of the scientist would be (a) since this provides us with credible evidence, whereas animal care-givers would probably answer (b) as they wish to see immediate implementation of anything that can improve animal welfare.

Resolving this dilemma is a complex situation and one that human society faces constantly in the field of medical science. Take the development of a drug to cure cancer; if one were discovered today it would probably be seven to ten years before such a drug would be being prescribed by doctors. The problem with this approach of empirical validation is that the time delay for environmental enrichment may only be a few months, but this time delay is sufficient to significantly demotivate animal care-givers. Clearly, a balance needs to be struck between the need for using only enrichment techniques that improve animal welfare and the need to motivate staff about animal welfare (see Chapter 6). As a compromise solution, I would suggest that if a technique is similar to one already validated (or validated on a closely-related species), then with some monitoring of the new enrichment (see Chapter 5 for example methodology), or 'rapid behavioural assessments', we can justify the implementation of the technique. Totally novel environmental enrichment techniques should always be empirically validated before being implemented.

The only creditable data we can have about the effect of environmental enrichment on animal welfare is from empirical studies designed using the scientific method. To simplify, to understand the effect of enrichment we must vary just one factor at a time (i.e. enriched condition versus the unenriched condition) having previously made control measurements before the one factor (enrichment) is varied (Martin & Bateson, 1993). Although we teach this in schools to children less than 10 years old, I never fail to be amazed by the number of environmental enrichment studies that vary several things simultaneously. For example, enriching the life of laboratory dogs by giving them a social companion, increasing their outside playtime, dietary change and the provision of toys. The problem with making sense of this example should be obvious; if we have found an effect we cannot determine which change or changes were responsible. Conceivably, we might find no effect since one form of enrichment might increase activity (e.g. outside playtime) and the other decrease activity (e.g. dietary change). To repeat, in empirical scientific studies of environmental enrichment we must vary only one thing at a time to establish its effect.

Once we have established the individual effects of social companionship, increasing outside playtime, dietary change and provision of toys, we can investigate the effects (and interactions) of these enrichments when provided simultaneously. Ideally, this would be done first as all pair-wise combinations, then all three-way combinations and finally all four enrichments simultaneously (a grand total of 14 treatment conditions including the original four enrichment conditions). In practice, most institutions will combine environmental enrichment conditions without first testing their combined effects.

Along with using a control and varying only one condition at a time, we need to decide whether to use the same subjects during the control and during the experimental manipulation, a 'within-subjects design'. The alternative is that we use matched (e.g. for age, sex etc.) but different subjects for the control and the enrichment, a 'between-subjects design' (Lehner, 1998). In general, environmental enrichment studies have tended to use a within-subjects design, often for the practical reason that fewer different subjects are required. Furthermore, the use of a within-subjects design allows us to use paired statistics (e.g. paired *t*-test, Wilcoxon matched-pairs test; Fowler *et al.*, 1998), that are effective in removing the effects of individual variation. An enrichment technique might have the effect of increasing exploratory behaviour in pet guinea pigs but some guinea pigs increase by 10% of their observation time and others by 70%. If we use a between-subjects design and appropriate statistical test (e.g., *t*-test or Mann-Whitney U test) then we would find no significant difference due to the variation in baseline- (control) and enrichment-condition levels of exploratory behaviour. Whereas, a within-subjects design and appropriate statistical test would detect that the exploratory behaviour of all guinea pigs was increasing, irrespective of individual differences. I am not denying the value of between-subject designs of experiments in the appropriate situation but given that environmental enrichment studies often have limited numbers of subjects whose characteristics may vary (e.g., age, sex, rearing history etc.), within-subject designs are in most cases more appropriate.

I do not intend to discuss the use of non-behavioural measures, such as physiological, to assess the effectiveness of environmental enrichment since such measures cannot be employed without proper staff training. Nor am I going to discuss in detail the use of behavioural tests, such as tonic immobility (a fear test) or Morris mazes (a spatial learning and memory test), instead, I refer the reader to Table 12.1 below (which cites the most common tests) and the references cited therein. Instead, I will briefly mention the commonly used behavioural recording methods.

Most environmental enrichment studies concern themselves with the changes in an animal's time budget. For example, during the enrichment period, does the animal spend more time playing and less time involved in abnormal behaviour? Time budget data can usually be collected by 'instantaneous time sampling' with a short time interval (ideally less than 30 seconds; Martin & Bateson, 1993). This means that the observer notes down the behaviour of the animal, according to a pre-written ethogram (list of behaviours) once every 30 seconds, on the exact time interval, for a set period of time (e.g. for one hour each day). If animals are housed in a group, the observer can use 'scan sampling' to record the behaviour of all animals at the same time, i.e. on the time interval the behaviour of each animal is observed quickly in succession and noted down. However, if the environmental enrichment study is concerned with using enrichment to improve social relationships between group members, or in measuring the increased complexity of a behaviour, different techniques are more appropriate. To analyse accurately and

Table 12.1 Commonly used behavioural assay tests.

Test Name	Measures	References
Emergence test	Fear	Grigor *et al.*, 1995b
Open-field	Fear	Clarke & Jones, 2000; Puppe *et al.*, 1999; Clausing *et al.*, 1997; Iuvone *et al.*, 1996
Novel object	Fear	Wemelsfelder *et al.*, 2000a
Tonic Immobility	Fear	Grigor *et al.*, 1995a; Mills & Faure, 2000 Jones, 1994; Jones & Waddington, 1992
Morris maze	Learning ability	Wainwright *et al.*, 1994; Hannigan *et al.*, 1993; Wainwright *et al.*, 1993; van Rijzingen *et al.*, 1997; Berman & Hannigan, 2000
Radial maze	Learning ability	Porsolt *et al.*, 1995; Macphail & Bolhuis, 2001; Hughes & Blight, 1999

understand social behaviour we require the full sequence of behaviour between participants. (This is like listening to someone talking on the telephone, we only hear one side of the conversation and it is difficult to understand exactly what is being said.) Thus, we need to record the behaviour of the animal(s) continuously for a set period of time, i.e. a full and accurate record of durations and frequencies of behaviour – this is called 'continuous recording'. The use of continuous recording often precludes the use of scan sampling since one observer cannot continuously record the behaviour of a whole group of animals. Instead, the observer usually records the behaviour of only one animal and the animal that it interacts with, this is called 'focal animal sampling'. The recording of the social behaviour of animals in large, physically-complex enclosures often requires the use of instantaneous and focal animal sampling.

12.2 Statistical Analysis

The only measure of credibility in scientific results comes from statistical proof. The problem with statistical analyses of data is that many people do not understand them and consequently it is easy to mislead someone. Huff (1991) has written a book called *How to Lie with Statistics* which contains wonderful examples of how the unknowledgeable person can be mislead by statistics. The problem with statistical tests is that they rely on the human operator to use them correctly and sensibly. Correct use depends on statistical knowledge, whereas sensible use depends on an understanding of the scientific field in which the statistics are being applied. A statistical test can show a statistically significant difference between two conditions (or treatments) but only the knowledgeable person can determine if such a difference is scientifically significant (or in our case, biologically significant). For example, the statistically significant difference in the percentage of time spent playing by pet guinea pigs on the baseline (control) compared to the enriched condition might only be 0.0001%, which is clearly biologically meaningless. These types of results tend to be generated when the data has top (i.e. all values are nearly maximal) or bottom (i.e. all values are nearly minimal or zero) effects (Lehner, 1998). Here I intend only to provide some basic advice on the use of statistics in environmental enrichment studies (the subject that I receive most communications about).

12.2.1 Non-parametric versus parametric tests

The field of statistics can be basically divided into tests that assume that the data to be analysed has a normal distribution – parametric statistics, or that the distribution of the data is essentially unknown – non-parametric statistics. Basically, parametric statistics work by comparing the means of different treatments, whereas non-parametric statistics work by comparing the medians of different treatments. Parametric statistics are in general more powerful than non-parametric statistics, they allow us to analyse data for complex effects, e.g. how do enrichment technique, age of the subjects, and sex of the subjects interact? However, to use parametric statistics we must first ascertain that our data meet certain requirements (e.g. the data are normally distributed) and if not we must use mathematical data transformations (e.g. square root the data) to achieve these requirements; this is unnecessary for non-parametric statistics. Thus, non-parametric statistics are far simpler to implement than parametric statistics. Also, for many parametric statistical tests there exists a non-parametric equivalent (see Table 12.2 for examples). Most people find non-parametric tests easier to use, therefore, I will focus on them in the rest of this chapter. Once a person becomes more confident in the use of non-parametric statistics, they may wish to use parametric statistics to analyse more complex designs of experiments. The final thing to mention is the difference between one-tailed and two-tailed statistical tests, such as the Wilcoxon matched pairs test. Normally, we use a two-tailed test, since we do not know if the behav-

Table 12.2 Commonly used statistical tests.

Parametric test	Non-parametric equivalent
Student's *t*-test	Mann-Whitney U-test
Matched *t*-test	Wilcoxon matched pairs test
One-way analysis of variance	Kruskal-Wallis test
Two-way analysis of variance	Friedmann's test
Pearson's correlation	Spearman rank correlation

iours we are measuring will increase or decrease. If, however, we had a strong reason to make a prediction that a behaviour would only increase (or decrease) then we could use a one-tailed test. (In general, with one-tailed tests a lower numerical level needs to be achieved to attain statistical significance. Thus, one could argue that the use of two-tailed tests is more statistically rigorous.)

12.2.2 Absolute versus proportional time budgets

Environmental enrichment must not just use up the animals' time in doing activities that humans prefer to observe, it should actually change the animals' motivation. Young and Lawrence (1996) demonstrated using a foraging device that manipulated the time budget of domestic pigs by altering the rate at which the pigs received food, demonstrating that we can occupy an animal's time budget with behaviour patterns that are essential to immediate survival. The increase in foraging reported by Young and Lawrence (1996) resulted in the significant decrease in resting and sleeping behaviour. Does this change in behaviour represent an improvement in the pigs' welfare? It has been suggested by Terlouw and Lawrence (1993) that only proportional changes in an animal's time budget are motivationally significant and thus related to animal welfare. I will illustrate by way of a theoretical example. Suppose the baseline daily time budget of free-range chickens is: 12 hours per day sleeping (locked in at night); 3 hours per day foraging; 3 hours per day socialising; and the remaining 6 hours are involved in abnormal behaviour. Now we introduce foraging enrichment (we scatter the hens' food around the field rather than placing it in a trough) and the time budget changes to: 12 hours per day sleeping; 5 hours per day foraging; 3 hours per day socialising; and the remaining 4 hours are involved in abnormal behaviour. The amount of time spent foraging has increased by 40% and the amount of time spent performing abnormal behaviour has decreased by a third. However, we need to consider that our hens had no choice but to spend 5 hours foraging and so the amount of time to perform other behaviours is reduced by the 2 hour increase and we also need to discount the 12 sleeping hours. Therefore, out of the non-sleeping hours the time outside of foraging behaviour has decreased to 7 hours per day and thus hens are performing abnormal behaviour for 57% of the available time. Before the foraging enrichment, the hens had 9 hours of non-foraging time of which 66% was spent performing abnormal behaviour. Thus, the proportional reduction, which relates more closely to motivational changes, has decreased much less (only 9%) than the absolute time budget (2 hours). We need to be careful, therefore, in the assessment of time budget changes, especially if the enriched behaviour pattern is one that relates to food or water intake. Theoretically, it is possible to use environmental enrichment to force an animal to forage all its waking hours and thereby totally eliminate the performance of abnormal behaviour but without decreasing the animal's motivation to perform abnormal behaviour.

12.2.3 Dealing with small sample sizes

In many cases we are confronted with undertaking a study of environmental enrichment with a small sample size (i.e. small number of individuals), this is especially the case in zoos (Saudargas & Drummer, 1996). Most statistical tests require a minimum of six individuals to function reliably. In the ideal world we would use 'power statistics' (see Fowler *et al.*, 1998) to determine our sample but often this is not possible due to practical constraints. How do we cope with small sample sizes, i.e. those less than six? A statistician would correctly tell you that no statistical analysis is possible because the power of a test to generalise to the whole population depends on the sample size used, i.e. number of individuals. (I should point out that nearly all statistical tests require that data points used in analysis be totally independent from one another.) The trick to overcome the computation problem but not the statistical problem of a small sample size is the use of pseudo-replication: this means representing the same individuals in the data set several times as if they were different individuals. For example, we could have an enrichment study with one animal that we observed for 8 hours per day for 10 days before enrichment (the baseline or control condition) and then watch it for an equal period of time during the enrichment condition. Normally, we would make an average for each behaviour for each case condition, i.e. each behaviour would have only two data points. It would be impossible to analyse such data; however, we could make an average per day and thereby increase our sample size to 10 data points for each treatment so analysis becomes possible. The results of this type of analysis involving pseudo-replication cannot be generalised to the whole captive population of our study animal. However, they can be used to determine whether enrichment has had a significant effect on the particular animal we have studied. The results of such a study on a rare and endangered species would be of value despite its small sample size.

The other trick that is used, and sometimes combined with pseudo-replication, is the pooling of a single group's data; statisticians refer to this as the 'pooling fallacy' (Fowler *et al.*, 1998). The behaviour of animals living in a group is not independent of other group members' behaviour, therefore, a group of animals (irrespective of group size) represents a sample size of one. It is possible to treat the behaviour of individual animals as if they were independent data points but as with pseudo-replication, this is not a correct statistical procedure and the conclusions that can be drawn from such results are limited (see above). I should stress that the use of pseudo-replication and pooling data should be last resorts when no other option is available since the results generated are applicable only to the animals tested.

12.2.4 Special behavioural indices

The empirical study of animal behaviour has a number of indices, which are used to provide numerical scores for behavioural expression. The most commonly used ones being indices of hierarchy and association (Martin & Bateson, 1993). In applied behaviour two other indices can also be used, the 'spread of participation index', which can measure the degree of enclosure utilisation (see Williams *et al.*, 1996), and the 'behavioural diversity index' (see Shepherdson *et al.*, 1993; Williams *et al.*, 1996), which measures what its name suggests.

12.3 Example Experimental Design and Associated Statistical Analyses

The following example uses a within-subjects ABA experimental design (A represents the first condition baseline and B represents the second condition enrichment); this is the design most commonly used in environmental-enrichment studies (e.g. Ings *et al.*, 1997). The experimental details for this study are as follows:

Experimental subjects: six primates (3 males and 3 females).
Housing: each animal is individually housed.
Enrichment: scatter feeding instead of bowl feeding.
Experimental design (ABA): baseline (A), enrichment (B) and post-enrichment (A).
Ethogram: resting, locomotion, foraging, abnormal, social call, other.
Sampling method: scan each cage once every 60 seconds and record behaviour.
Observation time: 20 hours for baseline, enrichment and post-enrichment.
Distribution of observations: 2 hours per day for 10 consecutive days.

Raw data are rarely collected on checksheets entered directly into the computer for analysis, unless we are interested in analysing the sequences of behaviour. Normally, the data are collated by animal and behaviour, as illustrated in Tables 12.3–12.5, and once in this format the data can be entered into the computer. This pre-collation of data before inputting to a computer is usually much more time efficient than entering raw data. Normally, I recommend either entering the data directly into the statistical software if it has a spreadsheet facility (Minitab has this

Table 12.3 Baseline (collated data, columns are total number of observation points).

Behaviour	M1	M2	M3	F1	F2	F3
Resting	240	252	264	228	276	264
Locomotion	360	348	336	372	324	336
Foraging	120	132	144	144	156	168
Abnormal	240	228	216	216	204	192
Social call	120	108	96	84	72	60
Other	120	132	144	156	168	180

M = Males and F = Females

Table 12.4 Enrichment (collated data, columns are total number of observation points).

Behaviour	M1	M2	M3	F1	F2	F3
Resting	180	192	204	168	216	204
Locomotion	420	408	396	432	384	396
Foraging	240	228	216	216	204	192
Abnormal	120	132	144	144	156	168
Social call	132	132	108	84	72	60
Other	108	108	132	156	168	180

Table 12.5 Post-enrichment (collated data, columns are total number of observation points).

Behaviour	M1	M2	M3	F1	F2	F3
Resting	252	268	252	240	268	252
Locomotion	348	336	348	360	336	348
Foraging	132	144	132	156	168	156
Abnormal	228	216	228	204	192	204
Social call	120	108	96	84	72	60
Other	120	132	144	156	168	180

Table 12.6 Summary statistics for 'Resting' behaviour (Table 12.3–12.5).

Experimental Period	Mean	Standard Deviation
Baseline	254	17.66
Enrichment	194	17.66
Post-enrichment	255	10.86

facility for example) or into a spreadsheet programme (e.g. Microsoft Excel) from which it can be cut and pasted into a statistical programme. Once all the data are entered into the computer we can start the statistical analysis. The first step is normally to produce some descriptive statistics, usually some measure of central tendency (e.g. mean or median) and some measure of variation (e.g. standard deviation or standard error of the mean) as illustrated in Table 12.6. Alternatively, you may prefer to make a visual representation of the data, e.g. frequency histograms.

The next step is to actually analyse the data; Figure 12.1 provides a flowchart summary of how we are going to analyse these data. Each behaviour for each animal in each experimental condition (i.e. 3 data points per animal and 18 in total) is analysed using a Kruskal-Wallis test with experimental condition (i.e. baseline, enrichment and post-enrichment) as the factor. The results of these analyses for resting behaviour are shown in Table 12.7. However, the Kruskal-

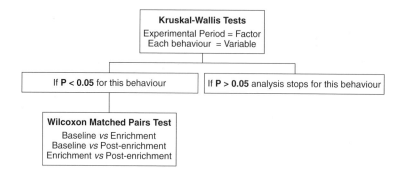

Figure 12.1 Flow-chart summary of a statistical analysis commencing with the Kruskal-Wallis test.

Table 12.7 Results of Wilcoxon Matched Pairs tests for 'Resting' behaviour (Table 12.3–12.5).

Matched Pairs	Wilcoxon Statistic	N	P
Baseline *vs* **Enrichment**	21	6	0.036*
Baseline *vs* **Post-enrichment**	8	6	0.675
Enrichment *vs* **Post-enrichment**	21	6	0.036*

*P < 0.05 (i.e. a statistically significant result)

Wallis test does not tell us where the significant difference(s) lie (i.e. are all conditions different from each other or only certain pairs), we need to use post-hoc Wilcoxon Matched Pairs test to discover this information (see Figure 12.1). The results of post-hoc testing for the behaviour 'Resting' are shown in Table 12.7. Here we can see that the significant differences are between the enrichment condition and the other two conditions. From Figure 12.2 and Table 12.6 we can see that the amount of time spent resting significantly decreased during the enrichment period in comparison with the baseline and the post-enrichment period. The opposite pattern would be seen for 'Foraging' behaviour (examine Tables 12.3–12.5).

I have of course presented highly stylised results. We may find that all the conditions are different from each other for a particular behaviour. If we discover a linear increase or decrease in behaviour across all three treatments, and hence across time, this suggests that a factor independent of enrichment causes the differences. For example, the song output of male birds may increase each day as spring commences and then start to decrease each day as autumn arrives. A number of studies have found that foraging enrichment results in an increase in foraging behaviour during enrichment and post-enrichment, i.e. the pair-wise significant differences are baseline versus enrichment and baseline versus post-enrichment (Shepherdson *et al.*, 1993; Williams *et al.*, 1996; Ings *et al.*, 1997). It has been suggested that this is the result of behavioural activation (Haskell *et al.*, 1996), the

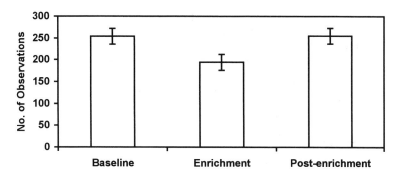

Figure 12.2 Results from a theoretical statistical analysis of the behaviour 'Resting'.

animal 'discovering' an outlet for its behaviour. In a famous case of behavioural activation, Morris (1964) describes how a serval that was fed a chicken with feathers on for the first time in its life, later indulged in an orgy of plucking; according to his description it plucked most of the grass in its enclosure.

It is of course possible to use more complex experimental designs for environmental enrichment. For example, Vick *et al.*, (2000) used a ABACAD design (A = Baseline, B = Enrichment simple, C = Enrichment responsive, D = Enrichment with food) with primates to try and disentangle the effects of food from other properties of an environmental enrichment device. I strongly warn against using an AB design (A = Baseline, B = Enrichment) because it does not allow us to discount the fact that behaviours may have been changing with time independent of the enrichment (see preceding paragraph). From personal experience I know that it is tempting to leave a successful enrichment technique in place but to do so scientifically weakens the study.

12.4 Has Animal Welfare been Improved?

Statistics, if correctly used, can only prove or disprove that there exists a difference between experimental conditions – the interpretation of the biological significance of these differences must be made by the experimenter. In Chapters 1 and 3 I have outlined the information that is needed to make such interpretations but it is up to the individual to make the interpretation and present it to the scientific community. It is only through scientific review and scrutiny that the individual's interpretation can be validated. I would, therefore, urge people to submit their studies for publication, even if the results are negative. The information in this chapter should hopefully encourage more people to conduct empirical studies of environmental enrichment and to analyse them statistically. If there is any doubt regarding statistical analyses, the advice of a professional statistician should be sought.

Information Sources about Environmental Enrichment

Living as we do in the information age where we are constantly bombarded with facts and figures, the risk of being overloaded with information is high. In this chapter I have tried to do two things for the reader, sieve through the ocean of information available and direct the reader to the best resources, and categorise resources as accurately as possible with commentaries on each resource. These two processes involve, of course, a personal choice and I am sure I have excluded a number of arguably worthy entries for which I apologise. In my defence, I can only say that I have recommended what I as an individual have found to be useful.

As in so many subjects related to animal welfare, people who work with environmental enrichment are incredibly generous in sharing their work. The following list of resources about environmental enrichment is the result of innumerable hours of work by the authors whose only reward is that they hope animal welfare can be improved by sharing information. I am grateful to the authors not only for their generosity but for making my life much easier. The quality of some of the internet databases, especially those of Reinhardt & Reinhardt (see below) is such that I have not needed to fill this book with examples.

13.1 Books

The availability of books on environmental enrichment for the different categories of animals is unfortunately patchy. For example, there are no books on environmental enrichment for farm or pet animals, a situation I hope that this book corrects. Here I have listed the books that I have found most useful in my experience of implementing enrichment, conducting enrichment studies and teaching about environmental enrichment. The list is by no means exhaustive and new books are appearing all the time. A final comment is that I have deliberately not included books which are only aimed at the specialist academic reader. The related subject of where to find information about a species to conduct an enrichment programme is a common one aimed at myself. The answer I give is that there now exist many excellent books about individual species or groups of related species, e.g. dolphins. These books are most easily found using the search engines of two internet-based bookshops: Amazon.com (*http://www.amazon.co.uk*) and the Natural History Book Club (*http://www.nhbs.co.uk*), using the species' common name as the keyword to search by.

It should be possible to borrow any of the books listed below from a public library but only by asking them to request a copy from a specialist library, such as the national library of your country. Depending on the country, this service may be free or, unfortunately, very expensive. As a fluent Brazilian Portuguese speaker I apologise for only recommending books in English but these are the best ones currently available.

ABWAK (1998) *Guidelines for Environmental Enrichment*. ed. David Field. Top Copy, Bristol.
These are multi-author guidelines written by a mixture of zoo professionals, including keepers, and scientists. The guidelines contain several chapters on theoretical and practical subjects but principally they cover the application of enrichment for nearly every existing animal group from fish to felids. Without hesitation I would say that these guidelines are a goldmine of tried and tested ways of enriching the lives of zoo animals and many of the ideas could also be applied to similar farm, laboratory and pet animals. The guidelines are presented in a ring binder to allow the reader to include some of their own material and to include new material when it is published in *Ratel* or other magazines. Thus, the guidelines are a living and growing document.

Appleby, M. C. & Hughes, B. O. (1997) *Animal Welfare*. CABI Publishing, Wallingford, Oxford (ISBN: 0851991807).
Probably the best introductory book on the subject of animal welfare available. The book is multi-authored and while its focus is farm animals, the theoretical concepts discussed within apply to any category of animal.

Bekoff, M. & Meaney, C. A. (1998) *Encyclopedia of Animal Rights and Animal Welfare*. Greenwood Press, Westport (ISBN: 0313299773).
An invaluable, if expensive, multi-author encyclopaedia that gives quick and highly accessible introductions to nearly all topics relating to animal rights and animal welfare.

Broom, D. M. & Johnson, K. G. (1993) *Stress and Animal Welfare*. Kluwer Academic Publishers, London & New York (ISBN: 0412395800).
A useful introduction to the subject of animal stress.

Dolins, F. L. (1999) *Attitudes to Animals: Views in Animal Welfare*. Cambridge University Press, Cambridge (ISBN: 052147342X).
A useful multi-author book with chapters on theoretical, educational and ethical issues relating to animal welfare.

Fraser, A. F. & Broom, D. M. (1996) *Farm Animal Behaviour and Welfare* (Third Edition). CABI Publishing, Wallingford, Oxford (ISBN: 0851991602).
A good basic text book that introduces the reader to basic information about farm animal welfare.

Kleiman, D. G., Allen, M. E., Thompson, K. V., Lumpkin, S. & Harris, H. (1996) *Wild Mammals in Captivity*. University of Chicago Press, Chicago (ISBN: 0226440036).
This multi-author book provides an excellent introduction to all subjects that pertain to the maintenance of captive mammals in zoos. It has particularly good sections on designing exhibits and on animal behaviour.

Lehner, P. (1998) *Handbook of Ethological Methods*. Cambridge University Press, Cambridge (ISBN: 0521637503).
The most comprehensive book available about how to study animal behaviour, covering everything from experimental design and recording methods to statistical analysis.

Markowitz, H. (1982) *Behavioral Enrichment in the Zoo*. Van Nostran Reinhold Co., New York (ISBN: 0442251254).
This was the first book published on environmental enrichment and while still interesting, its age shows. A book now primarily of historical interest.

Martin, P. & Bateson, P. (1993) *Measuring Behaviour*. Cambridge University Press, Cambridge (ISBN: 0521446147).
A must for anyone who is considering making a behavioural study about environmental enrichment. This concise little book is rightly the 'bible' for anyone interested in conducting behavioural research.

Shepherdson, D. J., Mellen, J. D. & Hutchins, M. (1998) *Second Nature*. Smithsonian Institution Press, Washington (ISBN: 1560983973).
This multi-author book consists of theoretical chapters about environmental enrichment in relation to zoos, some of which also provide useful examples of the application of environmental enrichment. The book is useful in teaching some theoretical concepts in relation to environmental enrichment but for animal care-givers needs to be supplemented with a book of examples and an introductory book on animal welfare.

UFAW (1995) *Environmental Enrichment Information Resources for Laboratory Animals*: 1965–1995. Universities Federation for Animal Welfare & Animal Welfare Information Centre, Wheathampstead (ISBN: 090076791X).
A comprehensive list of scientific papers for all major species of animals used in laboratories. Each species' section is introduced by a short article on environmental enrichment for that species by a scientific expert.

UFAW (1999) *Handbook on the Care and Management of Laboratory Animals*. Vol. 1 & 2. (ed. Trevor Poole), Blackwell Science, Oxford (ISBN: 0632051337).
The definitive guide to the care of laboratory animals, covering a wide range of species from the mouse to the octopus. The book is multi-authored, each author combining scientific knowledge with practical application, which is what makes this such an important book.

Warwick, C., Fyre, F. & Murphy, J. B. (1994) *Health and Welfare of Captive Reptiles*. Kluwer Academic Publishers, London & New York (ISBN: 0412550806).
One of the few books that concerns itself with the welfare of reptiles.

Wolfensohn, S. E. & Lloyd, M. H. (1998) *Handbook of Laboratory Animal Management and Welfare*. Blackwell Science, Oxford (ISBN: 0632050527).
A very useful introduction to the subject of laboratory animal management and welfare.

13.2 Pet Books

I have included this section on pet books due to the lack of information about environmental enrichment for this group of animals. The following books are compilations of ideas to enrich the lives of pet animals, however, I am not endorsing the ideas within these books, rather I am recommending them as a source of stimulation (which must be applied judiciously).

Delzio, S. & Ribarich, C. (1999) *Felinestein: Pampering the Genius in Your Cat*. Harper Collins, New York (ISBN: 0062736302).

Levchuk, H. (1994) *Doris Dingle's Crafty Cat Activity Book: Games, Toys & Hobbies to Keep Your Cat's Mind Active*. Alaska Northwest Books, Portland (ISBN: 1898697094).

Laland, S. (1994) *51 Ways to Entertain Your Housecat While You're Out*. Avon Books, New York (ISBN: 0380774313).

Walker, B. (2002) *The Cats' House*. Andrews McMeel Publishing, Kansas City (ISBN: 0740719254).

Reed, J. A. (1996) *The Whole Kitty Catalog: More than 800 Terrific Toys, Treats, and True Cat Facts for You and by Your Kitty*! Random House, London (ISBN: 0517886898).

Shems, E. (1998) *Totally Fun Things to Do with Your Cat (Play with Your Pet)*. John Wiley & Sons, Chichester & New York (ISBN: 0471195758).

Green, G. (2001) *The Cat & Dog Lovers' Idea Book*. Krause Publications, Iola (ISBN: 0873492161).

Haynes Rauen, S. (2000) *Sassy Cats: Purr-fect Craft Projects*. Martingale & Co Inc, Woodville (ISBN: 1564773280).

Rogers, L. (2000) *Cat Toys: How to Make Your Home a Feline Paradise*. Storey Country Wisdom Bulletin, A–251; Storey Books, North Adams (ISBN: 1580173004).

Cusick, D. (1997) *Cat Crafts: More Than 50 Purrfect Projects*. Sterling Publications, London (ISBN: 080699553X).

Crimmins, C. E. (1991) *Cat's Picnic: Greens, Games, and Guaranteed Fun for Your Favorite Feline*. Running Pr, Philadelphia (ISBN: 1561380504).

Rock, M. A. (1998) *Totally Fun Things to Do With Your Dog (Play With Your Pet)*. John Wiley & Sons, Chichester & New York (ISBN: 047119574X).

Ludwig, G. & Steimer, C. (1996) *Fun and Games With Your Dog: Expert Advice on a Variety of Activities for You and Your Pet*. Barrons Educational Series, Hauppauge (ISBN: 0812097211).

Fisher B. & Delzio, S. (1997) *Caninestein: Unleashing the Genius in Your Dog*. Harper Collins, New York (ISBN: 0062734857).

Kephart, P. (2000) *Housebound Dogs: How to Keep Your Stay-at-Home Dog Happy & Healthy*. Storey Country Wisdom Bulletin, A–270, Storey Books, North Adams (ISBN: 1580173624).

Jones, D. (1998) *Clicker Fun: Dog Tricks and Games Using Positive Reinforcement*. Howln Moon Press, Eliot (ISBN: 1888994088).

Hunter, R. (1997) *Fun and Games With Dogs: Educational and Fun Games to Teach Your Dog to Enjoy Working With You*. Howln Moon Press, Eliot (ISBN: 1888994002).

Borgenicht, J. & Borgenicht, M. (2001) *Doggy Days: Dozens and Dozens of Indoor and Outdoor Activities for You and Your Best Friend–Tricks and Games, Arts and Crafts, Stories and Songs*. Ten Speed Press, Berkeley (ISBN: 1580083234).

Athan, M. S. (2000) *Guide to a Well-Behaved Parrot*. Barrons Educational Series, Hauppauge (ISBN: 0764110306).

Athan, M. S. (2000) *Guide to Companion Parrot Behavior*. Barrons Educational Series, Hauppauge (ISBN: 0764106880).

Blanchard, S. (2000) *Companion Parrot Handbook*. PBIC Inc. (Pet Bird Information Council), Alameda (ISBN: 096712980X).

Somerville, B. & Bucsis, G. (2000) *Training Your Pet Rat*. Barrons Educational Series, Hauppauge (ISBN: 0764112082).

13.3 Journals

The following peer-reviewed journals often include empirical, experimental and theoretical articles on environmental enrichment. Such journals are aimed at the academic reader, such as undergraduate and above, and normally they are only freely available through a university library. However, it is often possible to get a photocopy of a specific article by making a request at a public library, the cost of course varies massively from country to country.

Animal Behaviour (Academic Press)
Principally, publishes papers on pure ethology with occasional papers on animal welfare and environmental enrichment; all categories of animals.

Animal Science (British Society of Animal Science)
Publishes the occasional paper on animal welfare or environmental enrichment; farm animals and horses.

Animal Welfare (UFAW)
Publishes many papers on animal welfare and environmental enrichment; all categories of animals.

Anthrozoos (Purdue University Press)
Publishes many papers on human–animal interactions and some on animal welfare related topics; principally pet animals.

Applied Animal Behaviour Science (Elsevier Science)
Publishes many papers on animal welfare and some on environmental enrichment; principally a farm animal journal.

Behaviour (Brill Academic Publishers)
The occasional paper on animal welfare but a good source of natural history-type ethological studies.

British Poultry Science (Carfax Publishing)
The occasional papers on animal welfare or environmental enrichment.

Contemporary Topics in Laboratory Animal Science (American Association of Laboratory Animal Science)

Frequently publishes papers on animal welfare and environmental enrichment – laboratory animals only.

Dodo (Jersey Wildlife Preservation Trust)
Publishes papers on behaviour and environmental enrichment; zoo animals only.

Ethology (Blackwell Wissenschafts-Verlag Gmbh.)
Publishes articles on animal behaviour and occasionally some on welfare related topics.

International Zoo Yearbook (Zoological Society of London)
Publishes articles on animal behaviour, welfare and environmental enrichment; zoo animals only.

Journal of Animal Science (American Association of Animal Science)
Publishes some articles on animal welfare and environmental enrichment; farm animals and horses only.

Journal of Applied Animal Welfare Sciences (Lawrence Erlbaum Associates Inc.)
Publishes papers on animal welfare and environmental enrichment; all categories of animals.

Journal of Medical Primatology (Munksgaard International Publications Ltd.)
Publishes the occasional paper on animal welfare or environmental enrichment; primates only.

Journal of Neurosciences (Society of Neuroscience)
Publishes the occasional paper on the neurological effects of environmental enrichment; articles principally use rodent models.

Lab Animal (Nature America Inc.)
Publishes some articles on animal welfare and environmental enrichment; laboratory animals only.

Laboratory Primate Newsletter (University of Madison, Wisconsin)
Frequently publishes articles on animal behaviour, animal welfare and environmental enrichment; laboratory housed primates only.

Physiology and Behavior (Pergamon-Elsevier Science Ltd.)
Publishes papers on animal behaviour, and occasionally some on animal welfare and environmental enrichment; principally laboratory studies using rodent models.

Poultry Science (Poultry Science Association Inc.)
Publishes the occasional paper on animal welfare or environmental enrichment; only farmed poultry.

Psychopharmacology (Springer-Verlag)
Publishes the occasional paper on the interaction between pharmacy and environmental enrichment; principally laboratory animal studies.

Zoo Biology (Wiley-Liss)
Frequently publishes papers on environmental enrichment, animal behaviour and animal welfare; only zoo animals.

13.4 Magazines

The following are non peer-reviewed magazines, therefore you need to scrutinise the studies they publish even more closely than those in peer-reviewed journals. They are aimed at the professional animal care-giver.

International Zoo News
Frequently publishes articles on animal behaviour, welfare and environmental enrichment. This magazine is an excellent source of news and information about zoos around the world; only zoo animals (*http://www.species.net*).

Ratel
Publishes many articles on animal welfare and environmental enrichment. The enrichment articles usually have been tested by a zoo keeper and as such are very practical but often they have not been studied systematically. The magazine is focussed on providing information to UK zoo keepers; only zoo animals (*http://www.abwak.org.uk*).

The Shape of Enrichment
The leading source of environmental enrichment ideas for zoo animals. Almost all articles are submitted by zoo keepers and therefore tend to be extremely practical but often they have not been studied systematically. This magazine is also an excellent source of information about conferences and news about environmental enrichment; only zoo animals (*http://www.enrichment.org*).

Zookeepers' Forum
Publishes many articles on animal welfare and environmental enrichment. The enrichment articles usually have been tested by a zoo keeper and as such are very practical but often they have not been systematically studied. The magazine is focussed on providing information for US zoo keepers; only zoo animals (*http://www.aazk.org*).

13.5 Organisations

The following is a list of organisations that are involved directly with animal welfare and some specifically with environmental enrichment. Most of these organisations will provide information about subjects within their remit to anyone who makes a formal request for information or at the very least will point you in the right direction. Many countries in the world have a government department concerned with animal well-being or non-governmental organisations (NGO) that advise on this subject. For the sake of brevity, I have not included these for every country but given examples mainly from the UK and the US. A good starting point in any country would be to contact the government department for farming, which usually has a section relating to animals. I have also not included any organisations that use political lobbying as a tool, such as animal rights groups, to increase the probability that the reader would receive unbiased information.

Animal Behaviour Society (ABS)

The professional society representing academics interested in animal behaviour and allied subjects, such as animal welfare in the Americas. The society co-publishes the journal *Animal Behaviour* with ASAB. It organises annual, themed conferences and has funds to assist members to present papers at conferences. The society also has funds to support small research projects (*http://www.animalbehavioursociety.com*).

American Zoo and Aquarium Association (AZA)

This organisation represents the interests of all major zoos in the US. It has specialist committees that focus on specific species and more general issues such as captive breeding. It has a specialist group whose focus is animal behaviour and environmental enrichment (*http://www.aza.org*).

Animal Procedures Committee (APC)

In the UK this is the Government's scientific advisory group on all issues, including welfare, that relate to laboratory animals. They frequently publish reports and make recommendations about welfare; only laboratory animals.

Animal Welfare Information Center (AWIC)

This centre is based in the US and its mission is to make information about animal welfare as widely available as possible. It has excellent links to US animal welfare information, laws and databases (*http://www.nal.usda.gov*).

Association for the Study of Animal Behaviour (ASAB)

The professional society representing academics interested in animal behaviour and allied subjects, such as animal welfare, in Europe and beyond. The society co-publishes the journal *Animal Behaviour* with ABS (which members receive at a very low cost). It organises annual, themed conferences and has funds to assist members to present papers at conferences. The society also has funds to support small research projects, including grants for undergraduates to undertake small scientific studies (*http://www.asab.org.uk*).

Association of British Wild Animal Keepers (ABWAK)

This organisation represents the interests of British zoo keepers; it publishes the magazine *Ratel* and other zoo related documents, such as the *Enrichment Guidelines*; it also organises occasional meetings (*http://www.abwak.org.uk*).

Institute of Animal Technicians (IAT)
This is the organisation that represents laboratory animal technicians in the UK. It provides training, reports and organises conferences which often have a section on environmental enrichment (*http://www.iat.org.uk*).

Companion Animal Welfare Council (CAWC)
In the UK this is the Government's scientific advisory group on all issues, including welfare, that relate to pet animals. They frequently publish reports and make recommendations about welfare; only pet animals (*http://www.cawc.org.uk*).

Farm Animal Welfare Council (FAWC)
In the UK this is the Government's scientific advisory group on all issues, including welfare, that relate to farm animals. They frequently publish reports and make recommendations about welfare; only farm animals (*http://www.fawc.org.uk*).

Federation of Zoos, Great Britain and Ireland
This is the organisation that represents most of the major zoos within the British Isles. It has a number of sub-committees including a research group that promote studies on zoo animal behaviour, welfare and environmental enrichment. It occasionally publishes articles and reports that relate to these topics. Also, it organises a conference once a year that often includes presentations on animal welfare related subjects; zoo animals only. Can be contacted through the Secretary, Zoological Gardens, Regent's Park, London, UK.

International Society of Applied Ethology (ISAE)
This society principally represents academics interested in animal welfare, the membership is dominated by those interested in farm animal welfare. The society organises annual conferences. Members are entitled to buy a subscription to the journal *Applied Animal Behaviour Science* at a greatly reduced price. It has an education committee (*http://www.isae.org.uk*).

Universities Federation for Animal Welfare (UFAW)
A unique organisation that promotes animal welfare through scientific research and its application. It publishes the journal *Animal Welfare*, for which members receive a reduced subscription, and many other reports and books that relate to animal welfare. It also funds scientific research (post-doctoral, PhD studentships and vacation scholarships for undergraduates) in the UK in welfare-related subjects. Also, it manages a number of sources of funding for the promotion of animal welfare. Its remit also includes the organising of occasional conferences and the provision of information to all types of institutions, governmental, scientific and public. Its work covers all types of animals (*http://www.ufaw.org.uk*). The postal address is: UFAW, The Old School, Brewhouse Hill, Wheathampstead, AL4 8AN, UK.

Zoos Forum
In the UK this is the government's scientific advisory group on all issues, including welfare, that relate to zoo animals. They frequently publish reports and make recommendations about welfare; only zoo animals (*http://www.defra.gov.uk*).

Zoo Outreach
This organisation is based in India and deals exclusively with trying to assist Indian zoos and the surrounding countries in increasing their animal-welfare standards. It also produces a newsletter in English about its work (*http://www.zooreach.org*).

13.6 Videos and Television

Widely available sources of information about enrichment are videos and television programmes. Many television programmes are available across the world albeit only on cable television.

Ask the Animals, Association for the Study of Animal Behaviour (ASAB) video.

Barking Mad, BBC television programme
This programme mainly covers behavioural problems that companion animals show and how to treat them, such as separation anxiety in dogs. Many of the experts also use enrichment as part of their solution to the behavioural problem. On many occasions this programme provides excellent ideas for the enrichment of household pets, a category of animal that has traditionally been ignored by their owners in terms of environmental enrichment. See the BBC web site for further information (*http://www.bbc.co.uk*).

The Shape of Enrichment video library
An ever-expanding library collection of videos on environmental enrichment for zoo animals. A few of the videos are available commercially but many are made in-house by US zoos. Many of the videos are excellent sources of ideas. The videos can be borrowed for the price of return postage. The video library has satellite offices in most continents, please see *The Shape of Enrichment* web site for details (*http://www.enrichment.org*).

Environmental Enrichment, Universities Federation for Animal Welfare (UFAW) video
A 40-minute long video available from UFAW (including a version translated into Brazilian Portuguese) that is divided into three sections: (1) an introduction to environmental enrichment; (2) examples of environmental enrichment in action; and (3) how to conduct an environmental enrichment study. Despite being more than 10 years old I still find this video to be an invaluable teaching tool for animal caregivers and university students. For further details of the video please see the UFAW web site (*http:www.ufaw.org.uk*).

Wild About Animals, Channel 4 television programme
A general television programme usually featuring one animal-welfare and often one environmental enrichment story per programme. The programme covers zoos,

pets and farm animals: I found it on occasion to be a useful source of ideas. See the Channel 4 website for further details (*http://www.channel4.co.uk*).

13.7 Information Resources on the World Wide Web

Having taught courses and workshops about environmental enrichment around the world I know that one of the best ways to share information quickly, cheaply and effectively is through the internet. Here I have listed some of the more useful web sites for environmental enrichment. Please be aware that internet addresses are, unfortunately, prone to changing, so if any of these prove inaccessible please accept my apologies.

The Web of Science (http://wos.mimas.ac.uk)
This is a database of scientific publications (1981–present) only accessible by scientists and university students in the UK (you need a username and password). It indexes over 17 million articles and it is possible to search the database for details of publications (i.e. author, title, year, journal, volume, pages) using keyword searches, such as 'environmental enrichment'. This is the database most academics turn to when searching for new articles about a subject.

Environmental Enrichment for Primates
(http://www.awionline.org/Lab_animals/biblio/enrich.htm)
This is a database of scientific papers developed by Victor and Annie Reinhardt on environmental enrichment for laboratory primates. The database can be searched using keywords, and the results include the full citation of found articles and sometimes their abstract.

Environmental Enrichment Scrapbook
(http://members.home.net/dscriv/index.html)
This is a collection of environmental enrichment ideas that have been submitted to this website which is maintained by Barnum-Scrivener.

Laboratory Primate Newsletter
(http://www.brown.edu/Research/Primate/enrich.html)
This is a database of complete articles on environmental enrichment and psychological well-being that have been published in *Laboratory Primate Newsletter*. The database is categorised into different areas such as group housing, toys etc. This is one of the best, easily accessible scientific resources about enrichment that is available.

The Shape of Enrichment (http://www.enrichment.org)
The website of the organisation and magazine of the same name. The website includes information about subscriptions to the magazine, writing articles for the

magazine, the International Conference on Environmental Enrichment, news and other information about environmental enrichment.

Maddie's Pet Adoption Center at the San Francisco SPCA
  (*http://www.sfspca.org/maddies.shtml*)
A website that demonstrates an immersion-type animal shelter that dogs and cats like in rooms that look like standard human living rooms rather than the classical bare cell.

CAUZ Network (http://www.selu.com/~bio/cauz/focus/focus07.html)
This network is primarily based in North America and is an association of scientists and zoo professionals. It has a group whose focus is environmental enrichment. The website has a database of contacts.

Environmental Enrichment for Laboratory Animals
  (*http://www.awionline.org/Lab_animals/biblio/refine.htm*)
This is a database of scientific papers developed by Victor and Annie Reinhardt on environmental enrichment for laboratory animals. The database can be searched using keywords and the results include the full citation of found articles and sometimes their abstract.

Environmental Enrichment Information Resources for Nonhuman Primates:
  1987–1992 (*http://netvet.wustl.edu/species/primates/primenv.txt*)
A list of references on this subject.

Environmental Enrichment for Farm Animals
  (*http://www.awionline.org/Lab_animals/biblio/lbfarm.htm*)
This is a database of scientific papers developed by Victor and Annie Reinhardt on environmental enrichment for farm animals. The database can be searched using keywords and the results include the full citation of found articles and sometimes their abstract.

Farm Animal Housing and Handling (http://www.grandin.com)
Professor Temple Grandin is a world expert on the design of housing for animals and on animal handling. Her website contains complete copies of many of her numerous articles which are often illustrated with excellent photos.

Canadian Council on Animal Care (http://www.ccac.ca/english/gublurb.htm)
Guidelines on animal welfare.

Primate Enrichment Forum (http://groups.yahoo.com/group/pef-list)
This is a discussion group's web site where members can exchange ideas and pick each others' brains about primate enrichment.

Tufts University (http://www.tufts.edu/vet/cfa/qol_bib.html)
References for enrichment in shelter animals.

Association of British Wild Animal Keepers (http://www.abwak.co.uk/enrich.htm)
Guidelines for environmental enrichment; a number of fully explained examples
of enrichment devices that are presented in the book of the same name (see above).

University of Wisconsin-Madison
(http://www.primatelit.library.wisc.edu/pin/pef/slide/intro.html)
Enrichment for caged rhesus macaques; a set of slides available to illustrate
laboratory primate enrichment.

Environmental Enrichment for Non-Human Primates
(http://www.awionline.org/Lab_animals/biblio/index.html)
An annotated bibliography for animal care personnel; a useful bibliography on
laboratory housed primates, especially those in the US, made available by David
Seelig, Victor and Annie Reinhardt.

Disney Enrichment (http://www.csew.com/enrich)
A site very useful for advice on planning and implementing environmental
enrichment.

Universities Federation for Animal Welfare (http://www.ufaw.org.uk)
A website with comprehensive links to all areas of animal welfare. Abstracts from
the journal *Animal Welfare* and full details of the huge range of animal welfare
activities that UFAW undertake are all available.

UK Home Office (http://www.homeoffice.gov.uk/new_indexs/index_anima.htm)
This site for laboratory animals includes all the UK's legal requirements for housing
animals in laboratories, plus many articles on related topics. It is also home to the
Animal Procedures Committee website.

UK Department for Environment, Food and Rural Affairs (Zoos)
(http://www.defra.gov.uk/wildlife-countryside/gwd/zoo.htm)
The UK Government's site for zoos; it contains copies of all laws pertaining to
zoos, it has links to the Zoos Forum and contains discussion documents about the
future of zoos in Europe.

UK Department for Environment, Food and Rural Affairs (farm animals)
(http://www.defra.gov.uk/animalh/welfare/publications/onfarm-gen.htm)
The UK Government's site dealing with farm animals; it is absolutely full of extremely useful information about farm animal health, welfare and legislation. It is
possible to download guidelines for the care and management of all farm-housed
species from this site. The site contains many other useful documents ready to be
downloaded. It is also home to the Farm Animal Welfare Councils website.

13.8 Enrichment Manuals, Lists and CD-ROMs

A number of zoos and laboratories around the world have now produced in-house
environmental enrichment manuals, some of which exist as paper copies and others

as CD-ROMS; this list is not meant to be exhaustive. The manuals usually consist of a paper on each type of enrichment, a full description (often with photographs) of the enrichment and an assessment of its usefulness by animal care-givers. Some of these manuals include literally hundreds of environmental enrichment techniques. It is my conviction that all institutions that manage animals should publish an environmental enrichment manual to demonstrate the seriousness with which they take animal welfare.

Copenhagen Zoo (Denmark) Environmental Enrichment Manual
This collection of ideas was produced by Bengt Holst. He can be contacted at the following address: Copenhagen Zoo, Sdr Fasanvej, Copenhagen, DK-2000 Frederiksberg, Denmark.

Metro Park Washington Zoo (USA)
David Shepherdson maintains a list of environmental enrichment. He can be contacted at the following address: Metro Washington Park Zoo, Portland 4001 S.W. Canyon Road, Portland, Oregon 97221–2799, USA.

Edinburgh Zoo (UK)
Gordon Mcleod has compiled into a manual all the environmental enrichment techniques used at Edinburgh Zoo. He can be contacted on: *gordon_mcleod@hotmail.com.*

Marwell Zoo (UK) Environmental Enrichment Manual
This manual is available on CD-Rom from the zoo.
(*http://www.marwell.org.uk/zr/enrichment/Enrich-CD-Main.htm*).

13.9 Conferences

Conferences are a great place to share your work with other people, discover new ideas (most research that is published is at least two years old) and to make contacts. While the price of attending a conference is often considerable, the benefits usually outweigh the costs. A number of professional organisations provide financial help for their members to present papers at conferences, e.g. ASAB.

International Conference on Environmental Enrichment
This conference is held in different locations around the world once every two years (on odd year numbers). The conference principally focuses on zoo animals with presentations ranging from zoo keepers to academic scientists in an attempt to blend practice and science together. Details of the conference and the possibilities to buy proceedings are listed on The Shape of Enrichment web site.

International Society of Applied Ethology
Has one international conference every year and a number of regional conferences every year (e.g. UK, Eastern Europe etc.) on applied behaviour or animal-welfare related subjects. Although the conferences often have a main theme they usually also include a session on free papers, i.e. a session for papers on any subject relat-

ing to animal welfare. It would be fair to say that these conferences are primarily attended by scientists interested in farm animals. Further details of the conferences can be found on the society's web site.

Laboratory Animal Conferences
Across the world many professional organisations representing laboratory animal technicians and scientists organise annual conferences which often include a section on subjects related to animal welfare. However, due to the persecution of such workers and scientists in various countries, the details of these conferences are known only to members of the organisations and obviously the conferences are open only to members of the organisation. This is a very sad but nonetheless necessary state of affairs.

13.10 Training Courses

A number of professionals in the field of environmental enrichment run training courses around the world when invited by specific organisations. These courses, however, are usually only available to professionals. A number professionals in the field also work as commercial consultants but many will work just for their expenses.

The American Zoo and Aquarium Association
The AZA group on behaviour and environmental enrichment run workshops in the USA; check the AZA web site for details.

The University of Edinburgh (UK)
Dr Natalie Waran runs short fee-paying courses on animal-welfare related topics in conjunction with Edinburgh Zoo, e.g. the international summer school on 'Zoo Animal Behaviour and Welfare'. Check the University of Edinburgh web site for details (*http://www.ed.ac.uk*).

The University of Cambridge (UK)
Professor Don Broom runs short fee-paying courses on animal welfare and related topics that are principally aimed at veterinary surgeons. Check the University of Cambridge web site for details (*http://www.cam.ac.uk*).

Active Environments Inc. (USA)
This commercial company runs fee-paying training courses in animal training and environmental enrichment but their expertise is primarily in animal training. Contact: Active Environments Inc., 7651 Santos Road, Lompoc, CA 93436, USA.

13.11 University Courses

Many degrees in zoology, biology and psychology have modules on animal behaviour, especially in European and North American universities. Some veterinary science courses now also include at least one module on animal welfare. A few specialist courses now exist that focus exclusively on animal behaviour and animal-welfare related subjects. Before registering for any course I would recommend that a prospective student checks the following details: (1) the module content (does the course deliver the subjects in which you are interested?); (2) the quality of the teaching (in the UK universities are given points out of 24 for teaching quality, 24 being high — most countries have systems of evaluating teaching quality); and (3) the quality of research (in the UK universities are given a score on a 1 to 5 scale, 5 being high — most countries have systems for evaluating teaching quality). The specialist courses I am familiar with and would recommend to students include:

BSc (Honours) Animal Science (Behaviour) and Animal Science (Welfare and Management) at the University of Lincoln, UK (*http://www.lincoln.ac.uk/lsa*). The course commences with the subjects fundamental to studying animal behaviour: biochemistry, anatomy, cell biology and physiology. The second year largely consists of modules in pure ethology and related subjects such as nutrition and reproduction. The final year is largely composed of animal welfare and applied animal behaviour modules. The final-year students also conduct a year-long research project.

MSc/Diploma Applied Animal Behaviour and Animal Welfare at the University of Edinburgh, UK (*http://www.ed.ac.uk*). This is undoubtedly the best post-graduate training course in the world available on the subject of animal welfare. Principally, the course is aimed at bioscience and veterinary science graduates who wish to specialise in applied behaviour and animal welfare. The course lasts 1 year, during which students study six modules about animal welfare and undertake a 5-month research project. Many of the graduates of this course have gone on to influential positions in animal-welfare organisations or into research.

13.12 Competitions

I think perhaps one of the most under-utilised motivators for the promotion of environmental enrichment is a competition for the best device, idea, enclosure etc. Such competitions are about promoting good work not just through the receipt of a prize but more from the positive publicity; I wish more institutions would set up such competitions around the world.

The Shape of Enrichment
Best paper submitted to the International Conference on Environmental Enrichment: international speakers are invited to submit their paper for consideration by a panel of experts that includes zoo keepers and scientists. The winner receives US$1000 towards the cost of attending the next conference.

Best designed environmental enrichment device: international candidates are invited to submit their design for an enrichment device that will be assessed by a panel of experts. The winner has his or her design constructed and receives a percentage of the profits.

See The Shape of Enrichment web site for details of both competitions (*http://www.enrichment.org*).

Universities Federation for Animal Welfare (UFAW)

Best new UK zoo animal exhibit: UK zoos are invited to submit the design of their new animal enclosures for evaluation in terms of animal welfare by a panel that includes zoo professionals and scientists. The winner receives a small cash prize and a plaque.

Best, cheap and practical new zoo environmental enrichment device: UK zoos are invited to submit the design of a new, cheap and practical environmental enrichment device for evaluation in terms of animal welfare by a panel that includes zoo professionals and scientists. The winner receives a small cash prize and a plaque.

See the UFAW web site for entry forms and further details of both competitions (*http:www.ufaw.org.uk*).

13.13 Suppliers

I do not intend to give a list of suppliers of enrichment equipment because the number of potential suppliers is enormous, and in each country the supplier is likely to have a different contact address. Also, most enrichment devices are not commercially available, they are made in-house, usually from things bought from DIY shops. The professional magazines and some journals for most types of animal care-givers contain adverts from companies that sell environmental enrichment devices. If you are looking for a commercially available product I would recommend that you check these sources of information first or contact a colleague in a similar institution.

13.14 End-note

I encourage all who work in environmental enrichment, individuals and organisations to make their information available to the global community by way of the internet. In my experience most animal keeping institutions and many individuals have access to information through the internet (even if it is only through a cybercafé), a medium which is both cheap and quick to update. The generosity of those individuals who provided the information cited above should be praised.

References

Anon. (1999) Animal welfare – RSPCA calls for tighter controls on pet trade. *Veterinary Record* **145**, p. 595.

Aengus, W. L. & Millam, J. R. (1999) Taming parent-reared orange-winged Amazon parrots by neonatal handling. *Zoo Biology* **18**, 177–87.

Ahola, L., Harri, M., Kasanen, S., Mononen, J. & Pyykonen, T. (2000) Effects of group housing in an enlarged cage system on growth, bite wounds and adrenal cortex function in farmed blue foxes (*Alopex lagopus*). *Animal Welfare* **9**, 403–12.

Aiello, L. C. & Dunbar, R. I. M. (1993) Neocortex size, group size, and the evolution of language. *Current Anthropology* **34**, 184–93.

Alberts, A. C. (1994) Dominance hierarchies in male lizards – implications for zoo management programs. *Zoo Biology* **13**, 479–90.

Alford, P. L., Bloomsmith, M. A., Keeling, M. E. & Beck, T. F. (1995) Wounding aggression during the formation and maintenance of captive, multimale chimpanzee groups. *Zoo Biology* **14**, 347–59.

Algers, B. & Jensen, P. (1991) Teat stimulation and milk production during early lactation in sows: effects of continuous noise. *Canadian Journal of Animal Science* **71**, 51–60.

Allen, M. E., Oftedal, O. T. & Baer, D. J. (1996) The feeding and nutrition of carnivores. In: *Wild Mammals in Captivity* (eds D. G. Kleiman, M. E. Allen, K. V. Thompson, S. Lumpkin & H. Harris), pp. 139–47. The University of Chicago Press, Chicago.

Ames, A. (1993) *The behaviour of captive polar bears*. UFAW, Wheathampstead.

Anderson, J. R. (1998) Social stimuli and social rewards in primate learning and cognition. *Behavioural Processes* **42**, 159–75.

Anderson, J. R. (1999) Primates and representations of self. *Cahiers de Psychologie Cognitive – Current Psychology of Cognition*, **18**, 1005–29.

Appleby, D. (1993) Separation anxiety in dogs. *Veterinary Record* **133**, p. 124.

Appleby, D. (1998) *Ain't Misbehavin'*. Broadcast Books, Bristol.

Appleby, M. C. (1997) Life in a variable world: behaviour, welfare and environmental design. *Applied Animal Behaviour Science* **54**, 1–19.

Appleby, M. C. & Hughes, B. O. (1997) *Animal Welfare*. CAB International, Cambridge.

Appleby, M. C. & Lawrence, A. B. (1987) Hunger as a cause of stereotypic behavior in tethered sows. *Applied Animal Behaviour Science* **17**, p. 377.

Appleby, M. C., Hughes, B. O. & Elson, H. A. (1992) *Poultry Production Systems: Behaviour, Management and Welfare*. CABI International, Oxford.

Archer, J. (1997) Why do people love their pets? *Evolution and Human Behavior* **18**, 237–59.

Arey, D. S. (1997) Behavioural observations of peri-parturient sows and the development of alternative farrowing accommodation: a review. *Animal Welfare* **6**, 217–29.

Arey, D. S. & Maw, S. J. (1995) Food substrates as environmental enrichment for pigs. *Farm Building Progress* **118**, 9–12.

Arnold, S. J. (1981) Behavioral variation in natural populations II. The inheritance of a feeding response in crosses between geographic races of the garter snake, *Thamnophis sirtalis*. *Evolution* **35**, 510–15.

Aruguete, M. S., Lyons, D. M., Mason, W. A. & Mendoza, S. P. (1998) Reactions of adult and immature squirrel monkeys to intergroup exposure. *Zoo Biology* **17**, 519–24.

Asheim, L. J. & Eik, L. O. (1998) The economics of fibre and meat on Norwegian dairy goats. *Small Ruminant Research* **30**, 185–90.

Askew, H. R. (1996) *Treatment of Behaviour Problems in Cats and Dogs*, Blackwell Publishing, Oxford.

Austen, C. (1994) *Rabbit Housing*. MSc thesis, University of Edinburgh, Scotland.

Baer, J. F. (1998) A veterinary perspective of potential risk factors in environmental enrichment. In: *Second Nature* (eds D. J. Shepherdson, J. D. Mellen & M. Hutchins), pp. 277–301. Smithsonian Institution Press, Washington.

Baker, K. C. (1997) Straw and forage material ameliorate abnormal behaviors in adult chimpanzees. *Zoo Biology* **16**, 225–36.

Ballou, J. D. & Foose, T. J. (1996) Demographic and genetic management of captive populations. In: *Wild Mammals in Captivity* (eds D. G. Kleiman, M. E. Allen, K. V. Thompson, S. Lumpkin & H. Harris), pp. 263–83. The University of Chicago Press, Chicago.

Balls, M. (1999) The funding of research on the three Rs in the EU. *Altex-Alternativen zu Tierexperimenten* **16**, 282–84.

Barbiers, R. B. (1985) Orangutans color preference for food items. *Zoo Biology* **4**, 287–90.

Barnes, C. A. & McNaughton, B. L. (1985) An age comparison of the rates of acquisition and forgetting in relation to long-term enhancement of the hippocampal synapses. *Behavioural Neuroscience* **99**, 1040–8.

Barnes, G. W. & Baron, A. (1961) Stimulus complexity and sensory reinforcement. *Journal of Comparative and Physiological Psychology* **54**, 466–9.

Barnett, J. L. & Newman, E. A. (1997) Review of welfare research in the laying hen and the research and management implications for the Australian egg industry. *Australian Journal of Agricultural Research* **48**, 385–402.

Barnett, J. L., Cronin, G. M., McCallum, T. H. & Newman, E. A. (1993) Effects of 'chemical intervention' techniques on aggression and injuries when grouping unfamiliar adult pigs. *Applied Animal Behaviour Science* **36**, 135–48.

Barrett, L., Dunbar, R. I. M. & Dunbar, P. (1992) Environmental influences on play-behavior in immature gelada baboons. *Animal Behaviour* **44**, 111–15.

Bauman, A. E., Russell, S. J., Furber, S. E. & Dobson, A. J. (2001) The epidemiology of dog walking: an unmet need for human and canine health. *Medical Journal of Australia* **175**, 632–4.

Baumgartner, G. (1994) Future developments and actual status of animal-welfare legislation. *Deutsche Tierarztliche Wochenschrift* **101**, 83–6.

Baumont, R. (1996) Palatability and feeding behaviour in ruminants. *Productions Animales* **9**, 349–58.

Baxter, E. & Plowman, A. B. (2001) The effect of increasing dietary fibre on feeding, rumination and oral stereotypies in captive giraffes (*Giraffa camelopardalis*). *Animal Welfare* **10**, 281–90.

Bayne, K., Dexter, S. & Strange, G. (1993) The effects of food provisioning and human interaction on the behavioural well-being of rhesus monkeys (*Macaca mulatta*). *Contemporary Topics in Laboratory Animal Science* **32**, 6–9.

Bazille, P. G., Walden, S. D., Koniar, B. L. & Gunther, R. (2001) Commercial cotton nesting material as a predisposing factor for conjunctivitis in athymic nude mice. *Lab Animal* **30**, 40–2.

Beattie, V. E., O'Connell, N. E., Kilpatrick, D. J. & Moss, B. W. (2000a) Influence of environmental enrichment on welfare-related behavioural and physiological parameters in growing pigs. *Animal Science* **70**, 443–50.

Beattie, V. E., O'Connell, N. E. & Moss, B. W. (2000b) Influence of environmental enrichment on the behaviour, performance and meat quality of domestic pigs. *Livestock Production Science* **65**, 71–9.

Beattie, V. E., Sneddon, I. A., Walker, N. & Weatherup, R. N. (2001) Environmental enrichment of intensive pig housing using spent mushroom compost. *Animal Science* **72**, 35–42.

Beattie, V. E., Walker, N. & Sneddon, I. A. (1996) An investigation of the effect of environmental enrichment and space allowance on the behaviour and production of growing pigs. *Applied Animal Behaviour Science* **48**, 151–8.

Beattie, V. E., Walker, N. & Sneddon, I. A. (1998) Preference testing of substrates by growing pigs. *Animal Welfare* **7**, 27–34.

Bekoff, M. (1997) Deep ethology, animal rights, and the great ape animal project: resisting speciesism and expanding the community of equals. *Journal of Agricultural & Environmental Ethics* **10**, 269–96.

Bell, D. D. & Adams, C. J. (1998) Environment enrichment devices for caged laying hens. *Journal of Applied Poultry Research* **7**, 19–26.

Bellaver, C. & Bellaver, I. H. (1999) Livestock production and quality of societies' life in transition economies. *Livestock Production Science* **59**, 125–35.

Bennett, A. T. D., Cuthill, I. C., Partridge, J. C. & Lunau, K. (1997) Ultraviolet plumage colors predict mate preferences in starlings. *Proceedings of the National Academy of Sciences of the United States of America* **94**, 8618–21.

Bennett, R. M. (1996) People's willingness to pay for farm animal welfare. *Animal Welfare* **5**, 3–11.

Bennett, R. M. (1997) Economics. In: *Animal Welfare* (eds M. C. Appleby & B. O. Hughes), pp. 235–48. CAB International, Cambridge.

Bennett, R. (1998) Measuring public support for animal welfare legislation: a case study of cage egg production. *Animal Welfare* 7, 1–10.

Beresford-Stoke, L. (1994) Free-ranging Primates in Zoos. MSc thesis, University of Edinburgh, Scotland.

Berger, B. G. (1996) Psychological benefits of an active lifestyle: what we know and what we need to know. *Quest* 48, 330–53.

Berman, R. E. & Hannigan, J. H. (2000) Effects of prenatal alcohol exposure on the hippocampus: spatial behavior, electrophysiology, and neuroanatomy. *Hippocampus* 10, 94–110.

Bernstein, P. L., Friedmann, E. & Malaspina, A. (2000) Animal-assisted therapy enhances resident social interaction and initiation in long-term care facilities. *Anthrozoos* 13, 213–24.

BHAG (1999) Behaviour and Husbandry Advisory Group, a scientific advisory group of the American Zoo and Aquarium Association Workshop at Disney's Animal Kingdom.

Biernaskie, J. & Corbett, D. (2001) Enriched rehabilitative training promotes improved forelimb motor function and enhanced dendritic growth after focal ischemic injury. *Journal of Neuroscience* 21, 5272–80.

Blake, E., Sherrit, D. & Skelton, T. (1998) Environmental enrichment of reptiles. In: *ABWAK's Guidelines for Environmental Enrichment* (ed. D. A. Field), pp. 43–9. Top Copy, Bristol.

Blakemore, C. & Mitchell, E. D. (1973) Environmental modification of the visual cortex and the neural basis of learning and memory. *Nature* 241, 467–8.

Bloomsmith, M. A. & Lambeth, S. P. (1995) Effects of predictable versus unpredictable feeding schedules on chimpanzee behavior. *Applied Animal Behaviour Science* 44, 65–74.

Bloomsmith, M. A. & Lambeth, S. P. (2000) Videotapes as enrichment for captive chimpanzees (*Pan troglodytes*). *Zoo Biology* 19, 541–51.

Bloomsmith, M. A., Brent, L. Y. & Schapiro, S. J. (1991) Guidelines for developing and managing an environmental enrichment program for nonhuman-primates. *Laboratory Animal Science* 41, 372–7.

Bloomsmith, M. A., Stone, A. M. & Laule, G. E. (1998) Positive reinforcement training to enhance the voluntary movement of group-housed chimpanzees within their enclosures. *Zoo Biology* 17, 333–41.

Bohnenkamp, G. (1994) *Help, My Dog has an Attitude.* James and Kenneth, Harpenden.

Boinski, S., Gross, T. S. & Davis, J. K. (1999a) Terrestrial predator alarm vocalizations are a valid monitor of stress in captive brown capuchins (*Cebus apella*). *Zoo Biology* 18, 295–312.

Boinski, S., Swing, S. P., Gross, T. S. & Davis, J. K. (1999b) Environmental enrichment of brown capuchins (*Cebus apella*): behavioral and plasma and fecal cortisol measures of effectiveness. *American Journal of Primatology* 48, 49–68.

Bollhofer, H. (1996) Animal welfare and profit motive in zoo pet shops compatible. *Deutsche Tierarztliche Wochenschrift* **103**, 65–6.

Bond, J. C. & Lindburg, D. G. (1990) Carcass feeding of captive cheetahs (*Acinonyx jubatus*): the effects of naturalistic feeding programs on oral health and psychological wellbeing. *Applied Animal Behaviour Science* **26**, 373–82.

Boness, D. J. (1996) Water quality management in aquatic mammal exhibits. In: *Wild Mammals in Captivity* (eds D. G. Kleiman, M. E. Allen, K. V. Thompson, S. Lumpkin & H. Harris), pp. 231–42. The University of Chicago Press, Chicago.

Borlongan, C. V. (2000) Motor activity-mediated partial recovery in ischemic rats. *Neuroreport* **11**, 4063–7.

Bostock, S. S. C. (1993) *Zoos and Animal Rights*. Routledge, London.

Brambell. (1965) *Report of the Technical Committee to Enquire into the Welfare of Animals kept Under Intensive Livestock Husbandry Systems*. Command Report 2836. Her Majesty's Stationary Office, London.

Brent, L. (1997) Behavioural management of nonhuman primates in a laboratory environment. In: *Proceedings of the Second International Conference on Environmental Enrichment* (ed. B. Holst), pp. 149–63. Copenhagen Zoo, Copenhagen.

Brent, L. & Belik, M. (1997) The response of group-housed baboons to three enrichment toys. *Laboratory Animals* **31**, 81–5.

Brent, L. & Eichberg, J. W. (1991) Primate puzzleboard – a simple environment enrichment device for captive chimpanzees. *Zoo Biology* **10**, 353–60.

Brent, L. & Stone, A. M. (1996) Long-term use of televisions, balls, and mirrors as enrichment for paired and singly caged chimpanzees. *American Journal of Primatology* **39**, 139–45.

Brent, L., Lee, D. R. & Eichberg, J. W. (1991) Evaluation of a chimpanzee enrichment enclosure. *Journal of Medical Primatology* **20**, 29–34.

Bride, I. (1998) Herpetofauna pet-keeping by secondary school students: causes for concern. *Society & Animals* **6**, 31–46.

Brodie, J. D. (1981) Health benefits of owning pet animals. *Veterinary Record* **109**, 197–9.

Brodie, S. J. & Biley, F. C. (1999) An exploration of the potential benefits of pet-facilitated therapy. *Journal of Clinical Nursing* **8**, 329–37.

Broom, D. M. (1999) Animal welfare: the concept of the issues. In: *Attitudes to Animals* (ed. F. Dolins), pp. 129–42. Cambridge University Press, Cambridge.

Broom, D. M. & Johnston, K. G. (1993) *Stress and Animal Welfare*. Kluwer Academic Publishers, Dordrecht.

Brooman, S. & Legge, D. (1997) *Law Relating to Animals*. Cavendish Publishing Ltd., London.

Brooman, S. & Legge, D. (2000) Animal welfare *vs* free trade – free trade wins: an examination of the animal welfare implications of R *v* Ministry of Agriculture, Fisheries and Food *ex p* Compassion in World Farming (1998). *Animal Welfare* **9**, 81–5.

Brown, C. & Laland, K. N. (2001) Social learning and life skills training for hatchery reared fish. *Journal of Fish Biology* **59**, 471–93.

Brown, C. S. & Loskutoff, N. M. (1998) A training program for noninvasive semen collection in captive western lowland gorillas (*Gorilla gorilla gorilla*). *Zoo Biology* **17**, 143–51.

Bubier, N. E. (1996) The behavioural priorities of laying hens: the effects of two methods of environment enrichment on time budgets. *Behavioural Processes* **37**, 239–49.

Buchanan-Smith, H. M. & Hardie, S. M. (1997) Tamarin mixed-species groups: an evaluation of a combined captive and field approach. *Folia Primatologica* **68**, 272–86.

Buchanan-Smith, H. M., Anderson, D. A. & Ryan, C. W. (1993). Responses of cotton-top tamarins (*Saguinus oedipus*) to faecal scents of predators and non-predators. *Animal Welfare* **2**, 17–32.

Burghardt, G. M., Ward, B. & Rosscoe, R. (1996) Problem of reptile play: environmental enrichment and play behavior in a captive nile soft-shelled turtle, *Trionyx triunguis*. *Zoo Biology* **15**, 223–38.

Burks, K. D., Bloomsmith, M. A., Forthman, D. L. & Maple, T. L. (2001) Managing the socialization of an adult male gorilla (*Gorilla gorilla gorilla*) with a history of social deprivation. *Zoo Biology* **20**, 347–58.

Burne, T. H. J., Murfitt, P. J. E. & Gilbert, C. L. (2000) Deprivation of straw bedding alters PGF(2 alpha)-induced nesting behaviour in female pigs. *Applied Animal Behaviour Science* **69**, 215–25.

Butterworth, A., Weeks, C. A., Crea, P. R. & Kestin, S. C. (2002) Dehydration and lameness in a broiler flock. *Animal Welfare* **11**, 89–94.

Byrne, R. W. (1999) Primate cognition: evidence for the ethical treatment of primates. In: *Attitudes to Animals* (ed. F. Dolins), pp. 114–25. Cambridge University Press, Cambridge.

Byrne, R. W. (2001) Evolution of primate cognition. *Cognitive Science* **24**, 543–70.

Byrne, R. W. & Whiten, A. (1988) Towards the next generation in data quality – a new survey of primate tactical deception. *Behavioral and Brain Sciences* **11**, 267–71.

Byrne, R. W., Corp, N. & Byrne, J. M. E. (2001) Estimating the complexity of animal behaviour: how mountain gorillas eat thistles. *Behaviour* **138**, 525–57.

Callard, M. D., Bursten, S. N. & Price, E. O. (2000) Repetitive backflipping behaviour in captive roof rats (*Rattus rattus*) and the effects of cage enrichment. *Animal Welfare* **9**, 139–52.

Campbell, W. (1995). *Owners Guide to Better Behavior in Dogs*. Alpine Publications, Loveland.

Capitanio, J. P. & Lerche, N. W. (1998) Social separation, housing relocation, and survival in simian AIDS: a retrospective analysis. *Psychosomatic Medicine* **60**, 235–44.

Cardiff, I. (1996) Assessing environmental enrichment for juvenile Jamaican boas (*Epicrates subflavus* Stejneger, 1901). *Dodo – Journal of the Wildlife Preservation Trusts* **32**, 155–62.

Carlstead, K. (1998) Determining the causes of stereotypic behaviour in zoo carnivores. In: *Second Nature* (eds D. J. Shepherdson, J. D. Mellen & M. Hutchins), pp. 172–83. Smithsonian Institution Press, Washington.

Carlstead, K. & Shepherdson, D. (1994) Effects of environmental enrichment on reproduction. *Zoo Biology* **13**, 447–58.

Carlstead, K., Brown, J. L. & Seidensticker, J. (1993) Behavioral and adrenocortical responses to environmental changes in leopard cats (*Felis-Bengalensis*). *Zoo Biology* **12**, 321–31.

Carlstead, K., Seidensticker, J. & Baldwin, R. (1991) Environmental enrichment for zoo bears. *Zoo Biology* **10**, 3–16.

Caro, T. M. (1994) *Cheetahs of the Serengeti Plains*. Chicago University Press, Chicago.

de Castro, J. M. (1988) The meal pattern of rats shifts from postprandial to preprandial when only five meals per day are scheduled. *Physiology & Behavior* **43**, 739–46.

Castro, M. I., Beck, B. B., Kleiman, D. G., Ruiz-Miranda, C. R. & Rosenberger, A. L. (1998) Environmental enrichment in reintroduction programs for golden lion tamarins (*Leontopithecus rosalia*). In: *Second Nature* (eds D. J. Shepherdson, J. D. Mellen & M. Hutchins), pp. 113–28. Smithsonian Institution Press, Washington.

Catlow, G. (1997) From sterile to stimulating: six years of management and husbandry changes to Edinburgh Zoo's monkey house. In: *Proceedings of the Second International Conference on Environmental Enrichment* (ed. B. Holst), pp. 205–8. Copenhagen Zoo, Copenhagen.

Catlow, G., Ryan, P. M. & Young, R. J. (1998) Please don't touch, we're being enriched! In: *Proceedings of the Third International Conference on Environmental Enrichment*. (eds V. J. Hare & K. Worley), pp. 209–17. Sea World, Orlando.

Chamove, A. S. (1986) Exercise improves behaviour: a rationale for occupational therapy. *British Journal of Occupational Therapy* **49**, 83–6.

Chamove, A. S. (1998) Electric fences for primates. *Laboratory Primate Newsletter* **37**, 12–14.

Chamove, A. S. & Anderson, J. R. (1989) Examining environmental enrichment. In: *Housing, Care and Psychological Well-being of Captive and Laboratory Primates* (ed. E. F. Segal), pp. 183–201. Noyes Publications, New Jersey.

Chamove, A. S. & Moodie, E. M. (1990) Are alarming events good for captive monkeys? *Applied Animal Behaviour Science* **27**, 169–76.

Chamove, A. S., Anderson, J. R., Morganjones, S. C. & Jones, S. P. (1982) Deep woodchip litter – hygiene, feeding, and behavioral enhancement in 8 primate species. *International Journal for the Study of Animal Problems* **3**, 308–18.

Chamove, A. S., Hosey, G. R. & Schaetzel, P. (1988) Visitors excite primates in zoos. *Zoo Biology* **7**, 359–69.

Chance, P. (1998) *Learning and Behavior*. Brooks/Cole, Berkley.

Chapillon, P., Manneche, C., Belzung, C. & Caston, J. (1999) Rearing environmental enrichment in two inbred strains of mice: 1. Effects on emotional reactivity. *Behavior Genetics* **29**, 41–6.

Charrassin, J. B., Bost, C. A., Putz, K., Lage, L., Dahier, T., Zorn, T. & Le Maho, Y. (1998) Foraging strategies of incubating and brooding king penguins, *Aptenodytes patagonicus*. *Oecologia* **114**, 194–201.

Cheal, M., Foley, K. & Kastenbaum, R. (1986) Brief periods of environmental enrichment facilitate adolescent development of gerbils. *Physiology & Behavior* **36**, 1047–51.

Chiszar, D., Radcliffe, C. W., Boyer, T. & Behler, J. L. (1987) Cover-seeking behavior in red spitting cobras (*Najamossambica pallida*) – effects of tactile cues and darkness. *Zoo Biology* **6**, 161–7.

Clarke, C. H. & Jones, R. B. (2000) Effects of prior video stimulation on open-field behaviour in domestic chicks. *Applied Animal Behaviour Science* **66**, 107–17.

Clark, G. I. & Boyer, W. N. (1993) The effects of dog obedience training and behavioral-counseling upon the human canine relationship. *Applied Animal Behaviour Science* **37**, 147–59.

Clausing, P., Mothes, H. K., Opitz, B. & Kormann, S. (1997) Differential effects of communal rearing and preweaning handling on open-field behavior and hot-plate latencies in mice. *Behavioural Brain Research* **82**, 179–84.

Clubb, R. & Mason, G. (1998) Foraging niche and stereotypic behaviour. In: *Proceedings of the 32nd Congress of the International Society of Applied Ethology* (eds I. Veissier & A. Boissy), pp. 174. International Society of Applied Ethology, Clermont-Ferrand.

Clutton-Brock, T. H., Gaynor, D., McIlrath, G. M., *et al.* (1999a) Predation, group size and mortality in a cooperative mongoose, *Suricata suricatta*. *Journal of Animal Ecology* **68**, 672–83.

Clutton-Brock, T. H., O'Riain, M. J., Brotherton, P. N. M., *et al.* (1999b) Selfish sentinels in cooperative mammals. *Science* **284**, 1640–44.

Cobb, S. C., Pope, S. K. & Williamson, R. (1995) Circadian rhythms to light–dark cycles in the lesser octopus, *Eledone cirrhosa*. *Marine and Freshwater Behaviour and Physiology* **26**, 47–57.

Cook, S. & Hosey, G. R. (1995) Interaction sequences between chimpanzees and human visitors at the zoo. *Zoo Biology* **14**, 431–40.

Cooper, J. J. & Appleby, M. C. (1997) Motivational aspects of individual variation in response to nestboxes by laying hens. *Animal Behaviour* **54**, 1245–53.

Cooper, J. J. & Mason, G. J. (2000) Increasing costs of access to resources cause re-scheduling of behaviour in American mink *Mustela vison*: implications for the assessment of behavioural priorities. *Applied Animal Behaviour Science* **66**, 135–51.

Cooper, J. J. & Nicol, C. J. (1991) Stereotypic behaviour affects environmental preference in bank voles (*Cletherionomys glareolus*). *Animal Behaviour* **41**, 971–7.

Cooper, J. J., McDonald, L. & Mills, D. S. (2000) The effect of increasing visual horizons on stereotypic weaving: implications for the social housing of stabled horses. *Applied Animal Behaviour Science* **69**, 67–83.

Corruccini, R. S. & Beecher, R. M. (1982) Occlusal variation related to soft diet in a nonhuman primate. *Science* **218**, 74–6.

Cotman, C. W. & Berchtold, N. C. (1998) Plasticity and growth factors in injury response. *Mental Retardation and Developmental Disabilities Research Reviews* **4**, 223–30.

Cox, C. (1987) Increase in the frequency of social interactions and the likelihood of reproduction among drills. In: *Proceedings of the American Association of Zoological Parks and Aquariums Annual Conference*, pp. 321–28. AAZPA, Wheeling.

Crockett, C. M. (1998) Psychological well-being of captive nonhuman primates: lessons from laboratory studies. In: *Second Nature* (eds D. J. Shepherdson, J. D. Mellen & M. Hutchins), pp. 129–52. Smithsonian Institution Press, Washington.

Crockett, C. M., Bowers, C. L., Bowden, D. M. & Sackett, G. P. (1994) Sex-differences in compatibility of pair-housed adult longtailed macaques. *American Journal of Primatology* **32**, 73–94.

Culik, B. M. & Wilson, R. P. (1995) Penguins disturbed by tourists. *Nature* **376**, 301–2.

Dahlqvist, P. M., Johansson, B. B., Risedal, A. *et al.* (2000) NGFI-A and NGFI-B mRNA expression correlates with improved functional recovery induced by environmental enrichment after middle cererbral artery occlusion in rats. *Stroke* **31**, p. 338.

Dahlqvist, P., Zhao, L., Johansson, I. M. *et al.* (1999) Environmental enrichment alters nerve growth factor-induced gene A and glucocorticoid receptor messenger RNA expression after middle cerebral artery occlusion in rats. *Neuroscience* **93**, 527–35.

Damm, B. I., Vestergaard, K. S., Schroder-Petersen, D. L. & Ladewig, J. (2000) The effects of branches on prepartum nest building in gilts with access to straw. *Applied Animal Behaviour Science* **69**, 113–24.

Davis, H. & Balfour, A. D. (1992) *The Inevitable Bond: Examining Scientist–Animal Interactions.* Cambridge University Press, Cambridge.

Davis, N. J., Prescott, N. B., Savory, C. J. & Wathes, C. M. (1999) Preferences of growing fowls for different light intensities in relation to age, strain and behaviour. *Animal Welfare* **8**, 193–203.

Dawkins, M. S. (1983) Battery hens name their price: consumer demand theory and the measurements of ethological 'needs'. *Animal Behaviour* **31**, 1195–205.

Dawkins, M. S. (1990) From an animal's point of view: motivation, fitness and animal welfare. *Behavioural and Brain Sciences* **13**, 1–61.

Day, J. E. L., Spoolder, H. A. M., Burfoot, A., Chamberlain, H. L. & Edwards, S. A. (2002) The separate and interactive effects of handling and environmental enrichment on the behaviour and welfare of growing pigs. *Applied Animal Behaviour Science* **75**, 177–92.

DeLeon, I. G., Anders, B. M., Rodriguez-Catter, V. & Neidert, P. L. (2000) The effects of noncontingent access to single-versus multiple-stimulus sets on self-injurious behavior. *Journal of Applied Behavior Analysis* **33**, 623–6.

DenOuden, M., Nijsing, J. T., Dijkhuizen, A. A. & Huirne, R. B. M. (1997) Economic optimization of pork production-marketing chains. 1. Model input on animal welfare and costs. *Livestock Production Science* **48**, 23–37.

Desmond, T. & Laule, G. (1994) Use of positive reinforcement training in the management of species for reproduction. *Zoo Biology* **13**, 471–7.

De Vleeschouwer, K., Leus, K., Van Elsacker, L. (2003) Stability of breeding and non-breeding groups of golden-headed lion tamarins (*Leontopithecus chysomelas*). *Animal Welfare* **12**, 251–68.

Dodman, N. (1997) *The Cat Who Cried for Help.* Bantham, New York.

Duffy, S. N., Craddock, K. J., Abel, T. & Nguyen, P. V. (2001) Environmental enrichment modifies the PKA-dependence of hippocampal LTP and improves hippocampus-dependent memory. *Learning & Memory* **8**, 26–34.

Dunbar, R. I. M. (1983a) Structure of gelada baboon reproductive units. 2. Social relationships between reproductive females. *Animal Behaviour* **31**, 556–64.

Dunbar, R. I. M. (1983b) Structure of gelada baboon reproductive units. 3. The male's relationship with his females. *Animal Behaviour* **31**, 565–75.

Dunbar, R. I. M. (1983c) Structure of gelada baboon reproductive units. 4. Integration at group level. *Zeitschrift Für Tierpsychologie – Journal of Comparative Ethology*, **63**, 265–82.

Dunbar, R. I. M. (1992) Neocortex size as a constraint on group-size in primates. *Journal of Human Evolution* **22**, 469–93.

Dunbar, R. I. M. (1995) Neocortex size and group-size in primates – a test of the hypothesis. *Journal of Human Evolution* **28**, 287–96.

Dunbar, R. I. M. (1998) The social brain hypothesis. *Evolutionary Anthropology* **6**, 178–90.

Dunbar, R. I. M. & Bever, J. (1998) Neocortex size predicts group size in carnivores and some insectivores. *Ethology* **104**, 695–708.

Dunbar, R. I. M. & Dunbar, E. P. (1981) The grouping behavior of male walia ibex with special reference to the rut. *African Journal of Ecology* **19**, 251–63.

Dunbar, R. I. M. & Dunbar, P. (1988) Maternal time budgets of gelada baboons. *Animal Behaviour* **36**, 970–80.

Duncan, I. J. H. (1978) The interpretation of preference tests in animal behaviour. *Applied Animal Ethology* **4**, 197–200.

Duncan, I. J. H. (1996) Animal welfare defined in terms of feelings. *Acta Agriculturae Scandinavica* Section a–Animal Science, 29–35.

Duncan, I. J. H. & Fraser, D. (1997) Understanding animal welfare. In: *Animal Welfare* (eds M. C. Appleby & B. O. Hughes), pp. 19–31. CAB International, Cambridge.

Duncan, I. J. H. & Petherick, J. C. (1991) The implications of cognitive-processes for animal-welfare. *Journal of Animal Science* **69**, 5017–22.

Eddy, T. J., Gallup, G. G. & Povinelli, D. J. (1996) Age differences in the ability of chimpanzees to distinguish mirror-images of self from video images of others. *Journal of Comparative Psychology*, **110**, 38–44.

Edney, A. T. B. (1988) *The Waltham Book of Cat and Dog Nutrition*. Pergamon Press Ltd, Oxford.

Eichberg, J. W., Lee, D. R., Butler, T. M., Kelley, J. & Brent, L. (1991) Construction of playgrounds for chimpanzees in bio-medical research. *Journal of Medical Primatology* **20**, 12–16.

Eisenberg, J. F. (1981) *The Mammal Radiations*. University of Chicago Press, Chicago.

Elfadil, A. A., Vaillancourt, J. P. & Duncan, I. J. H. (1998) Comparative study of body characteristics of different strains of broiler chickens. *Journal of Applied Poultry Research* **7**, 268–72.

Embury, A. S. (1997) Planting for environmental enrichment at Melbourne Zoo. In: *Proceeding of the Second International Conference on Environmental Enrichment* (ed. B. Holst), pp. 290–8. Copenhagen Zoo, Copenhagen.

Epple, G., Mason, J. R., Aronov, E. *et al.* (1995) Feeding responses to predator-based repellents in the mountain beaver (*Aplodontia rufa*). *Ecological Applications* **5**, 1163–70.

Erkert, H. G. (1989) Lighting requirements of nocturnal primates in captivity – a chronobiological approach. *Zoo Biology* **8**, 179–91.

Escorihuela, R. M., Fernandezteruel, A., Tobena, A. *et al.* (1995) Early environmental stimulation produces long-lasting changes on beta-adrenoceptor transduction systems. *Neurobiology of Learning and Memory* **64**, 49–57.

Escorihuela, R. M., Tobena, A. & Fernandezteruel, A. (1994) Environmental enrichment reverses the detrimental action of early inconsistent stimulation and increases the beneficial effects of postnatal handling on shuttlebox learning in adult rats. *Behavioural Brain Research* **61**, 169–73.

Estep, D. Q. & Baker, S. C. (1991) The effects of temporary cover on the behavior of socially housed stumptailed macaques (*Macaca arctoides*). *Zoo Biology* **10**, 465–72.

Evans, M. (2001) Environmental enrichment for pet parrots. *In Practice* **23**, 596–8.

Fagen, R. (1992) Play, fun, and communication of well-being. *Play & Culture* **5**, 40–58.

Farm Animal Welfare Council (1992) FAWC updates the five freedoms. *The Veterinary Record* **131**, 357.

Farrell, R., Evans, S. & Corbett, D. (2001) Environmental enrichment enhances recovery of function but exacerbates ischemic cell death. *Neuroscience* **107**, 585–92.

Ferchmin, P. A., Bennett, E. L. & Rosenzweig, M. R. (1975) Direct contact with enriched environment is required to alter cerebral weights in rats. *Journal of Comparative and Physiological Psychology* **88**, 360–7.

Fernandez-Teruel, A., Escorihuela, R. M., Castellano, B., Gonzalez, B. & Tobena, A. (1997) Neonatal handling and environmental enrichment effects on emotionality, novelty/reward seeking, and age-related cognitive and hippocampal impairments: focus on the Roman rat lines. *Behavior Genetics* **27**, 513–26.

Fischbacher, M. & Schmid, H. (1999) Feeding enrichment and stereotypic behavior in spectacled bears. *Zoo Biology* **18**, 363–71.

Fitch, H. M. & Fagan, D. A. (1982) Focal paletine erosion associated with dental malocclusion in captive cheetahs. *Zoo Biology* **4**, 295–310.

Flannigan, G. & Dodman, N. H. (2001) Risk factors and behaviors associated with separation anxiety in dogs. *Journal of the American Veterinary Medical Association* **219**, 460–6.

Flint, M. & Murray, P. J. (2001) Lot-fed goats – the advantages of using an enriched environment. *Australian Journal of Experimental Agriculture* **41**, 473–6.

Fogle, B. (1994) *The Complete Dog Training Manual*. Dorling Kindersley, London.

Forthman-Quick, D. L. (1984) An integrative approach to environmental engineering in zoos. *Zoo Biology* **3**, 65–78.

Forthman-Quick, D. L. (1998) Toward optimal care for confined ungulates. In: *Second Nature* (eds D. J. Shepherdson, J. D. Mellen & M. Hutchins), pp. 236–61. Smithsonian Institution Press, Washington.

Foster, T. C. & Dumas, T. C. (2001) Mechanism for increased hippocampal synaptic strength following differential experience. *Journal of Neurophysiology* **85**, 1377–83.

Fowler, J., Cohen, L. & Jarvis, P. (1998) *Practical Statistics for Field Biology*. Wiley, Chichester.

Frame, L. H., Malcom, J. R., Frame, G. W. & van Lawick, H. (1979) Social organisation of African wild dogs (*Lycaon pictus*) on the Serengeti plains, Tanzania 1967–1978. *Zeitschrift für Tierpsychologie – Journal of Comparative Ethology* **50**, 225–49.

Fraser, D. & Duncan, I. J. H. (1998) 'Pleasures', 'pains' and animal welfare: toward a natural history of affect. *Animal Welfare* 7, 383–96.

Fraser, D. & Matthews, L. R. (1997) Preference and motivation testing. In: *Animal Welfare* (eds M. C. Appleby & B. O. Hughes), pp. 159–73. CAB International, Cambridge.

Fraser, D., Weary, D. M., Pajor, E. A. & Milligan, B. N. (1997) A scientific conception of animal welfare that reflects ethical concerns. *Animal Welfare* 6, 187–205.

Fregonesi, J. A. & Leaver, J. D. (2001) Behaviour, performance and health indicators of welfare for dairy cows housed in strawyard or cubicle systems. *Livestock Production Science* 68, 205–16.

Fritz, J., Howell, S. M. & Schwandt, M. L. (1997) Colored light as environmental enrichment for captive chimpanzees (*Pan troglodytes*). *Laboratory Primate Newsletter* 36, 1–4.

Gagne, J., Gelinas, S., Martinoli, M. G. *et al.* (1998) AMPA receptor properties in adult rat hippocampus following environmental enrichment. *Brain Research* 799, 16–25.

Galef, B. G. (1976) The social transmission of acquired behaviour: a discussion of tradition and social learning in vertebrates. *Advances in the Study of Behavior* 6, 77–100.

Garner, P. W., Rennie, K. M. & Miner, J. L. (1996) Sharing attention to toys: adolescent mother–toddler dyads. *Early Development & Parenting* 5, 101–10.

Garrett, C. M. & Smith, B. E. (1994) Perch color preference in juvenile green tree pythons, *Chondropython viridis*. *Zoo Biology* 13, 45–50.

Goldfoot, D. A. (1977) Rearing conditions which support or inhibit later sexual potential of laboratory-born rhesus monkeys: hypotheses and diagnostic behaviors. *Laboratory Animal Science* 27, 548–56.

Gomez-Pinilla, F., So, V. & Kesslak, J. P. (1998) Spatial learning and physical activity contribute to the induction of fibroblast growth factor: neural substrates for increased cognition associated with exercise. *Neuroscience* 85, 53- 61.

Goodall, J. (1986) *The Chimpanzees of Gombe – Patterns of Behaviour*. Belknap Press of Harvard University, Massachusetts.

Greer, E. R., Diamond, M. C. & Tang, J. M. W. (1981) Increase in thickness of cerebral-cortex in response to environmental enrichment in brattleboro rats deficient in vasopressin. *Experimental Neurology* 72, 366–78.

Gregory, N. G. (2000) Consumer concerns about food. *Outlook on Agriculture* 29, 251–7.

Grigor, P. N., Hughes, B. O. & Appleby, M. C. (1995a) Effects of regular handling and exposure to an outside area on subsequent fearfulness and dispersal in domestic hens. *Applied Animal Behaviour Science* 44, 47–55.

Grigor, P. N., Hughes, B. O. & Appleby, M. C. (1995b) Emergence and dispersal behavior in domestic hens – effects of social rank and novelty of an outdoor area. *Applied Animal Behaviour Science* 45, 97–108.

Grigor, P. N., Hughes, B. O. & Appleby, M. C. (1995c) Social inhibition of movement in domestic hens. *Animal Behaviour* 49, 1381–8.

Grindrod, J. A. E. & Cleaver, J. A. (2001) Environmental enrichment reduces the performance of stereotypic circling behaviour in captive common seals (*Phoca vitulina*). *Animal Welfare* 10, 53–63.

Grinnell, J. & McComb, K. (1996) Maternal grouping as a defense against infanticide by males: evidence from field playback experiments on African lions. *Behavioral Ecology* **7**, 55–9.

Grinnell, J. & McComb, K. (2001) Roaring and social communication in African lions: the limitations imposed by listeners. *Animal Behaviour* **62**, 93–8.

de Groot, J., de Jong, I. C., Prelle, I. T. & Koolhaas, J. M. (2000) Immunity in barren and enriched housed pigs differing in baseline cortisol concentration. *Physiology & Behavior* **71**, 217–23.

Gunnar, M. R. (1980) Control, warning signals, and distress in infancy. *Developmental Psychology* **16**, 281–9.

Gvaryahu, G., Cunningham, D. L. & Vantienhoven, A. (1989) Filial imprinting, environmental enrichment, and music application effects on behavior and performance of meat strain chicks. *Poultry Science* **68**, 211–17.

Hahn, N. E., Lau, D., Eckert, K. & Markowitz, H. (2000) Environmental enrichment-related injury in a macaque (*Macaca fascicularis*): intestinal linear foreign body. *Comparative Medicine* **50**, 556–8.

Hamm, R. J., Temple, M. D., O'Dell, D. M., Pike, B. R. & Lyeth, B. G. (1996) Exposure to environmental complexity promotes recovery of cognitive function after traumatic brain injury. *Journal of Neurotrauma* **13**, 41–7.

Hancocks, D. (1971) Animals and Architecture. Praeger, New York.

Hancocks, D. (1996) The design and use of moats and barriers. In: *Wild Mammals in Captivity* (eds D. G. Kleiman, M. E. Allen, K. V. Thompson, S. Lumpkin & H. Harris), pp. 191–203. The University of Chicago Press, Chicago.

Hanlon, R. T., Forsythe, J. W. & Joneschild, D. E. (1999) Crypsis, conspicuousness, mimicry and polyphenism as antipredator defences of foraging octopuses on Indo-Pacific coral reefs, with a method of quantifying crypsis from video tapes. *Biological Journal of the Linnean Society* **66**, 1–22.

Hannigan, J. H., Berman, R. F. & Zajac, C. S. (1993) Environmental enrichment and the behavioral-effects of prenatal exposure to alcohol in rats. *Neurotoxicology and Teratology* **15**, 261–6.

Hansen, L. T. & Berthelsen, H. (2000) The effect of environmental enrichment on the behaviour of caged rabbits (*Oryctolagus cuniculus*). *Applied Animal Behaviour Science* **68**, 163–78.

Harcourt, R. (1991) The development of play in the South-American fur-seal. *Ethology* **88**, 191–202.

Harri, M., Lindblom, J., Malinen, H. *et al.* (1999) Effect of access to a running wheel on behavior of C57BL/6J mice. *Laboratory Animal Science* **49**, 401–5.

Harrison, R. (1964) *Animal Machines*. Vincent Stuart Ltd., London.

Hart, L. A. (1994) The Asian elephants – driver partnership: the drivers' perspective. *Applied Animal Behaviour Science* **40**, 297–312.

Hartung, J. (2000) Some aspects of animal welfare in livestock production. *Deutsche Tierarztliche Wochenschrift* **107**, 503–6.

Harvey, N. C., Preston, K. L. & Leete, A. J. (1996) Reproductive behavior in captive Californian condors (*Gymnogyps californianus*). *Zoo Biology* **15**, 115–25.

Haskell, M. J. & Hutson, G. D. (1996) The pre-farrowing behaviour of sows with access to straw and space for locomotion. *Applied Animal Behaviour Science* **49**, 375–87.

Haskell, M. J., Terlouw, E. M. C., Lawrence, A. B. & Erhard, H. W. (1996) The relationship between food consumption and persistence of post-feeding foraging behaviour in sows. *Applied Animal Behaviour Science* **48**, 249–62.

Hassmen, P., Koivula, N. & Uutela, A. (2000) Physical exercise and psychological wellbeing: a population study in Finland. *Preventive Medicine* **30**, 17–25.

Hawthorne, A. J., Loveridge, G. G. & Horrocks, L. J. (1997) The behaviour of domestic cats in response to a variety of surface textures. In: *Proceedings of the Second International Conference on Environmental Enrichment* (ed. B. Holst), pp. 84–94. Copenhagen Zoo, Copenhagen.

Hayes, K. T., Feistner, A. T. C. & Halliwell, E. C. (1996) The effect of contraceptive implants on the behavior of female Rodrigues fruit bats, *Pteropus rodricensis*. *Zoo Biology* **15**, 21–36.

Headey, B. (1999) Health benefits and health cost savings due to pets: preliminary estimates from an Australian national survey. *Social Indicators Research* **47**, 233–43.

Healy, S. D. & Tovée, M. J. (1999) Environmental enrichment and impoverishment: neurophysiological effects. In: *Attitudes to Animals* (ed. F. Dolins), pp. 54–76. Cambridge University Press, Cambridge.

Hebert, P. L. & Bard, K. (2000) Orang-utan use of vertical space in an innovative habitat. *Zoo Biology* **19**, 239–51.

Hediger, H. (1950) *Wild Animals in Captivity*. Butterworths, London.

Hediger, H. (1955) *The Psychology and Behaviour of Animals in Zoos and Circuses*. Butterworths, London.

Hediger, H. (1969) *Man and Animal in the Zoo*. Routledge and Kegon Paul, London.

van Heezik, Y. & Seddon, P. J. (2001) Influence of group size and neonatal handling on growth rates, survival, and tameness of juvenile houbara bustards. *Zoo Biology* **20**, 423–33.

Heidbrink, G. A. (1997) Incorporating alternative materials into the enhancement of primary housing areas. In: *Proceedings of the Second International Conference on Environmental Enrichment* (eds B. Holst), pp. 95–102. Copenhagen Zoo, Copenhagen.

Hemsworth, P. H. & Barnett, J. L. (1987) Human–animal interactions. *Veterinary Clinics of North America – Food Animal Practice* **3**, 339–56.

Hemsworth, P. H. & Gonyou, H. W. (1997) Human Contact. In: *Animal Welfare* (eds M. C. Appleby & B. O. Hughes), pp. 205–17. CAB International, Cambridge.

Hemsworth, P. H., Barnett, J. L., Beveridge, L. & Matthews, L. R. (1995) The welfare of extensively managed dairy-cattle – a review. *Applied Animal Behaviour Science* **42**, 161–82.

Hemsworth, P. H., Coleman, G. J., Barnett, J. L. & Borg, S. (2000) Relationships between human–animal interactions and productivity of commercial dairy cows. *Journal of Animal Science* **78**, 2821–31.

Henderson, J. V. & Waran, N. K. (2001) Reducing equine stereotypies using an Equiball (TM). *Animal Welfare* **10**, 73–80.

Hill, D. A. (1999) Effects of provisioning on the social behaviour of Japanese and rhesus macaques: implications for socio-ecology. *Primates* **40**, 187–98.

Hill, R. A. & Dunbar, R. I. M. (1998) An evaluation of the roles of predation rate and predation risk as selective pressures on primate grouping behaviour. *Behaviour* **135**, 411–30.

van Hoek, C. S. & King, C. E. (1997) Causation and influence of environmental enrichment on feather picking of the crimson-bellied conure (*Pyrrhura perlata perlata*). *Zoo Biology* **16**, 161–72.

Holmes, S. N., Riley, J. M., Juneau, P., Pyne, D. & Hofing, G. L. (1995) Short-term evaluation of a foraging device for non-human Primates. *Laboratory Animals* **29**, 364–9.

Holst, B. (1997) Introduction to the environmental enrichment program in Copenhagen Zoo. In: *Proceedings of the Second International Conference on Environmental Enrichment* (eds B. Holst), pp. 244–50. Copenhagen Zoo, Copenhagen.

Holst, B. (1998) The ethics of environmental enrichment. In: *Proceedings of the Third International Conference on Environmental Enrichment* (eds V. J. Hare & K. E. Worley), pp. 45–8. The Shape of Enrichment, San Diego.

Hoplight, B. J., Sherman, G. F., Hyde, L. A. & Denenberg, V. H. (2001) Effects of neocortical ectopias and environmental enrichment on Hebb-Williams maze learning in BXSB mice. *Neurobiology of Learning and Memory* **76**, 33–45.

Horrell, R. I., A'Ness, P. J., Edwards, S. A. & Eddison, J. C. (2001) The use of nose-rings in pigs: consequences for rooting, other functional activities, and welfare. *Animal Welfare* **10**, 3–22.

Hosey, G. R. (2000) Zoo animals and their human audiences: what is the visitor effect? *Animal welfare* **9**, 343–57.

Hosey, G. R. & Druck, P. L. (1986) The influence of zoo visitors on the behaviour of captive primates. *Applied Animal Behaviour Science* **18**.

Houpt, K., Houpt, T. R., Johnson, J. L., Erb, H. N. & Yeon, S. C. (2001) The effect of exercise deprivation on the behaviour and physiology of straight stall confined pregnant mares. *Animal Welfare* **10**, 257–67.

Houser, W. D., Reinhardt, V., Cowley, D., Eisele, S. & Vertein, R. (1987) Socializing individually caged, female rhesus monkeys for the purpose of environmental enrichment. *Laboratory Animal Science* **37**, 509.

Howkins, A. & Merricks, L. (2000) 'Dewy-eyed-veal-calves': live animal exports and middle-class opinion, 1980–1995. *Agricultural History Review* **48**, 85–103.

Hsia, L. C. & Wood-Gush, D. G. M. (1984) The temporal patterns of food intake and allelomimetic feeding by pigs of different ages. *Animal Ethology* **11**, 271–82.

Hubrecht, R. C. (1993) A comparison of social and environmental enrichment methods for laboratory housed dogs. *Applied Animal Behaviour Science* **37**, 345–61.

Huff, D. (1991) *How to lie with statistics*. Penguin Books, London.

Hughes, B. O. (1996) FAWC's 'five freedoms'. *Veterinary Record* **138**, 651.

Hughes, B. O. & Duncan, I. J. H. (1988) The notion of ethological need, models of motivation and animal-welfare. *Animal Behaviour* **36**, 1696–707.

Hughes, R. N. & Blight, C. M. (1999) Algorithmic behaviour and spatial memory are used by two intertidal fish species to solve the radial maze. *Animal Behaviour* **58**, 601–13.

Hullar, I., Fekete, S., Andrasofszky, E., Szocs, Z. & Berkenyi, T. (2001) Factors influencing the food preference of cats. *Journal of Animal Physiology and Animal Nutrition* **85**, 205–11.

Humphrey, N. K. (1976) The social function of intellect. In: *Growing Points in Ethology* (eds P. P. G. Bateson & R. A. Hinde), pp. 303–17. Cambridge University Press, Cambridge.

Hunter, E. J., Jones, T. A., Guise, H. J., Penny, R. H. C. & Hoste, S. (2001) The relationship between tail biting in pigs, docking procedure and other management practices. *Veterinary Journal* **161**, 72–9.

Hurst, J. L., Barnard, C. J., Hare, R., Wheeldon, E. B. & West, C. D. (1996) Housing and welfare in laboratory rats: time-budgeting and pathophysiology in single-sex groups. *Animal Behaviour* **52**, 335–60.

Hutchins, M. R., Gordon, I. J., Kyriazakis, I. & Jackson, F. (2001) Sheep avoidance of faeces-contaminated patches leads to a trade-off between intake rate of forage and parasitism in subsequent foraging decisions. *Animal Behaviour* **62**, 955–64.

Hutchins, M., Hancocks, D. & Crockett, C. M. (1984) Naturalistic solutions to the problems of captive animals. *Zoologische Garten* **54**, 28–42.

Ickes, B. R., Pham, T. M., Sanders, L. A., Albeck, D. S., Mohammed, A. H. & Granholm, A. C. (2000) Long-term environmental enrichment leads to regional increases in neurotrophin levels in rat brain. *Experimental Neurology* **164**, 45–52.

Illius, A. W. & Gordon, I. J. (1993) Diet selection in mammalian herbivores: constraints and tactics. (ed. R. N. Hughes), pp. 157–81. Blackwell Science, Oxford.

Inglis, I. R. & Ferguson, N. J. K. (1986) Starlings search for food rather than eat freely available, identical food. *Animal Behaviour* **34**, 614–16.

Inglis, I. R., Forkman, B. & Lazarus, J. (1997) Free food or earned food? A review and fuzzy model of contrafreeloading. *Animal Behaviour* **53**, 1171–91.

Inglis, I. R., Langton, S., Forkman, B. & Lazarus, J. (2001) An information primacy model of exploratory and foraging behaviour. *Animal Behaviour* **62**, 543–57.

Ings, R., Waran, N. K. & Young, R. J. (1997) Attitude of zoo visitors to the idea of feeding live prey to zoo animals. *Zoo Biology* **16**, 343–7.

Ings, R., Waran, N. K. & Young, R. J. (1997) Effect of wood-pile feeders on the behaviour of captive bush dogs (*Speothos venaticus*). *Animal Welfare* **6**, 145–52.

Iuvone, L., Geloso, M. C. & DellAnna, E. (1996) Changes in open field behavior, spatial memory, and hippocampal parvalbumin immunoreactivity following enrichment in rats exposed to neonatal anoxia. *Experimental Neurology* **139**, 25–33.

Jagoe, A. & Serpell, J. (1996) Owner characteristics and interactions and the prevalence of canine behaviour problems. *Applied Animal Behaviour Science* **47**, 31–42.

Jensen, M. B. & Kyhn, R. (2000) Play behaviour in group-housed dairy calves, the effect of space allowance. *Applied Animal Behaviour Science* **67**, 35–46.

Jensen, M. B., Vestergaard, K. S. & Krohn, C. C. (1998) Play behaviour in dairy calves kept in pens: the effect of social contact and space allowance. *Applied Animal Behaviour Science* **56**, 97–108.

Joffe, J. M., Rawson, R. A. & Mulick, J. A. (1973) Control of their environment reduces emotionality in rats. *Science* **180**, 1383–4.

Johannesson, T. & Sorensen, J. T. (2000) Evaluation of welfare indicators for the social environment in cattle herds. *Animal Welfare* 9, 297–316.

Johansson, B. B. (1996) Functional outcome in rats transferred to an enriched environment 15 days after focal brain ischemia. *Stroke* 27, 324–6.

Johansson, B. B. & Belichenko, P. V. (2002) Neuronal plasticity and dendritic spines: effect of environmental enrichment on intact and postischemic rat brain. *Journal of Cerebral Blood Flow and Metabolism* 22, 89–96.

Jones, R. B. & Waddington, D. (1992) Modification of fear in domestic chicks, *Gallus gallus domesticus*, via regular handling and early environmental enrichment. *Animal Behaviour* 43, 1021–33.

Jones, R. B. (1994) Regular handling and the domestic chicks fear of human beings – generalization of response. *Applied Animal Behaviour Science* 42, 129–43.

de Jong, I. C., Prelle, I. T., van de Burgwal, J. A. *et al.* (2000a) Effects of environmental enrichment on behavioral responses to novelty, learning, and memory, and the circadian rhythm in cortisol in growing pigs. *Physiology & Behavior* 68, 571–8.

de Jong, I. C., Prelle, I. T., van de Burgwal, J. A. *et al.* (2000b) Effects of rearing conditions on behavioural and physiological responses of pigs to preslaughter handling and mixing at transport. *Canadian Journal of Animal Science* 80, 451–8.

Kamphues, J. (1993) Nutritionally caused disturbances in companion birds – reasons, influences, tasks. *Monatshefte für Veterinarmedizin* 48, 85–90.

Kastelein, R. A. & Wiepkema, P. R. (1988) The significance of training for the behaviour of stellar sea lions (*Eumetopias jubata*) in human care. *Aquatic Mammals* 14, 39–41.

Kastelein, R. A. & Wiepkema, P. R. (1989) A digging trough as occupational therapy for pacific walrusses (*Odobenus rosmarus divergens*) in human care. *Aquatic Mammals* 15, 9–17.

Keeling, L. J. & Duncan, I. J. H. (1991) Social spacing in domestic fowl under seminatural conditions – the effect of behavioral activity and activity transitions. *Applied Animal Behaviour Science* 32, 205–17.

Kells, A., Dawkins, M. S. & Borja, M. C. (2001) The effect of a 'freedom food' enrichment on the behaviour of broilers on commercial farms. *Animal Welfare* 10, 347–56.

Kelly, H. R. C., Bruce, J. M., Edwards, S. A., English, P. R. & Fowler, V. R. (2000) Limb injuries, immune response and growth performance of early-weaned pigs in different housing systems. *Animal Science* 70, 73–83.

Kessel, A. & Brent, L. (2001) The rehabilitation of captive baboons. *Journal of Medical Primatology* 30, 71–80.

King, N. E. & Mellen, J. D. (1994) The effects of early experience on adult copulatory-behavior in zoo-born chimpanzees (*Pan troglodytes*). *Zoo Biology* 13, 51–9.

Kingston, S. G. & Hoffman-Goetz, L. (1996) Effect of environmental enrichment and housing density on immune system reactivity to acute exercise stress. *Physiology & Behavior* 60, 145–50.

Kitchener, A. (1991) *The Natural History of the Wild Cats*. Comstock, New York.

Kitchener, A. C. (1999) Watch with mother: a review of social learning in the Felidae. In: *Mammalian Social Learning: Comparative and Ecological Perspectives* (eds H. O. Box & K. R. Gibson), pp. 236–58. Cambridge University Press, Cambridge.

Kleiman, D. G. (1994) Mammalian sociobiology and zoo breeding programs. *Zoo Biology* **13**, 423–32.

Klont, R. E., Hulsegge, B., Hoving-Bolink, A. H. *et al.* (2001) Relationships between behavioral and meat quality characteristics of pigs raised under barren and enriched housing conditions. *Journal of Animal Science* **79**, 2835–43.

Knierim, U. & Jackson, W. T. (1997) Legislation. In: *Animal Welfare* (eds M. C. Appleby & B. O. Hughes), pp. 249–64. CAB International, Cambridge.

Kohn, B. (1994) Zoo animal-welfare. *Revue Scientifique et Technique de l'Office International des Epizooties* **13**, 233–45.

Kono, H., Reid, P. J. & Kamil, A. C. (1998) The effect of background cuing on prey detection. *Animal Behaviour* **56**, 963–72.

Korte, S. M. (2001) Corticosteroids in relation to fear, anxiety and psychopathology. *Neuroscience and Biobehavioral Reviews* **25**, 117–42.

Korthals, M. (2001) Taking consumers seriously: two concepts of consumer sovereignty. *Journal of Agricultural & Environmental Ethics* **14**, 201–15.

Kratochvil, H. & Schwammer, H. (1997) Reducing acoustic disturbances by aquarium visitors. *Zoo Biology* **16**, 349–53.

Krebs, J. R. & Davies, N. B. (1987) *An Introduction to Behavioural Ecology.* Blackwell Scientific Publications, Oxford.

Kreger, M. D. & Mench, J. A. (1993) Physiological and behavioral-effects of handling and restraint in the ball python (*Python regius*) and the blue-tongued skink (*Tiliqua scincoides*). *Applied Animal Behaviour Science* **38**, 323–36.

Kreger, M. D., Hutchins, M. & Fascione, N. (1998) Context, ethics, and environmental enrichment in zoos and aquariums. In: *Second Nature* (eds D. J. Shepherdson, J. D. Mellen & M. Hutchins), pp. 59–82. Smithsonian Institution Press, Washington.

Krohn, C. C., Jago, J. G. & Boivin, X. (2001) The effect of early handling on the socialisation of young calves to humans. *Applied Animal Behaviour Science* **74**, 121–33.

Krohn, T. C., Ritskes-Hoitinga, J. & Svendsen, P. (1999) The effects of feeding and housing on the behaviour of the laboratory rabbit. *Laboratory Animals* **33**, 101–7.

Kuehler, C., Kuhn, M., Kuhn, J. E., Lieberman, A., Harvey, N. & Rideout, B. (1996) Artificial incubation, hand-rearing, behavior, and release of common 'Amakihi (*Hemignathus virens virens*): surrogate research for restoration of endangered Hawaiian forest birds. *Zoo Biology* **15**, 541–53.

Kuhnen, G. (1999) Housing-induced changes in the febrile response of juvenile and adult golden hamsters. *Journal of Experimental Animal Science* **39**, 151–5.

Kundera, M. (1984) *The Unbearable Lightness of Being.* Faber & Faber, London.

Lambeth, S. P. & Bloomsmith, M. A. (1992) Mirrors as enrichment for captive chimpanzees (*Pan troglodytes*). *Laboratory Animal Science* **42**, 261–6.

Lambeth, S. P., Bloomsmith, M. A. & Alford, P. L. (1997) Effects of human activity on chimpanzee wounding. *Zoo Biology* **16**, 327–33.

Lantermann, W. (1997) Parrots and 'their' people – Deficits of a relationship. *Praktische Tierarzt* **78**, 470–71.

Law, G. & Tatner, P. (1998) Behaviour of a captive pair of clouded leopards (*Neofelis nebulosa*): introduction without injury. *Animal Welfare* **7**, 57–76.

Law, G., Boyle, H., Johnson, J. & Macdonald, A. (1990) Food presentation: bears. *Ratel* **17**, 103–5.

Law, G., MacDonald, A. & Reid, A. (1997) Dispelling some common misconceptions about the keeping of felids in captivity. *International Zoo Yearbook* **35**, 197–207.

Law, G., MacDonald, A. & Reid, A. (1998) Enrichment of felids. In: *ABWAK Guidelines for Environmental Enrichment* (ed. D. A. Field), pp. 109–32. Top Copy, Bristol.

Lawrence, A. B. & Rushen, J. (1993) Stereotypic animal behaviour. CAB International, Wallingford.

Le Magnen, J. (1985) *Hunger.* Cambridge University Press, Cambridge.

Lea, S. E. G. & Dittrich, W. H. (1999) What do birds see in moving video images? *Cahiers de Psychologie Cognitive – Current Psychology of Cognition* **18**, 765–803.

Lehner, P. N. (1998) *Handbook of Ethological Methods.* Cambridge University Press, Cambridge.

Lemercier, H. (2000) Environmental enrichment: music, day and dusk, how do they influence the rat's behaviour in laboratory (*Rattus norvegicus*)? *Sciences et Techniques de l'Animal de Laboratoire* **25**, 23–30.

Lemon, W. C. & Barth, R. H. (1992) The effects of feeding rate on reproductive success in the zebra finch, *Taeniopygia guttata. Animal Behaviour* **44**, 851–7.

Levoy, B. (1998) Pet ownership brings proven health benefits. *Veterinary Economics* **39**, p. 16.

Lewis, K. P. (2000) A comparative study of primate play behaviour: implications for the study of cognition. *Folia Primatologica* **71**, 417–21.

Lidfors, L. (1997) Behavioural effects of environmental enrichment for individually caged rabbits. *Applied Animal Behaviour Science* **52**, 157–69.

Lindberg, A. C. & Nicol, C. J. (1997) Dustbathing in modified battery cages: is sham dustbathing an adequate substitute? *Applied Animal Behaviour Science* **55**, 113–28.

Lindburg, D. G. (1988) Improving the feeding of captive felids through the application of field data. *Zoo Biology* **7**, 211–18.

Line, S. W., Morgan, K. N. & Markowitz, H. (1991) Simple toys do not alter the behavior of aged rhesus monkeys. *Zoo Biology* **10**, 473–84.

Lomas, C. A., Piggins, D. & Phillips, C. J. C. (1998) Visual awareness. *Applied Animal Behaviour Science* **57**, 247–57.

van Loo, P. L. P., Kruitwagen, C. L. J. J., Van Zutphen, L. F. M., Koolhaas, J. M. & Baumans, V. (2000) Modulation of aggression in male mice: influence of cage cleaning regime and scent marks. *Animal Welfare* **9**, 281–95.

Loveridge, G. G. (1998) Environmentally enriched dog housing. *Applied Animal Behaviour Science* **59**, 101–13.

Lowen, C. & Dunbar, R. I. M. (1994) Territory size and defendability in primates. *Behavioral Ecology and Sociobiology* **35**, 347–54.

Ludes-Fraulob, E. & Anderson, J. R. (1999) Behaviour and preferences among deep litters in captive capuchin monkeys (*Cebus capucinus*). *Animal Welfare* **8**, 127–34.

Lukas, K. E., Hamor, G., Bloomsmith, M. A., Horton, C. L. & Maple, T. L. (1999) Removing milk from captive gorilla diets. The impact on regurgitation and reingestion (R/R) and other behaviors. *Zoo Biology* **18**, 515–28.

Lund, J. D. & Jorgensen, M. C. (1999) Behaviour patterns and time course of activity in dogs with separation problems. *Applied Animal Behaviour Science* **63**, 219–36.

Lutz, C. K. & Novak, M. A. (1995) Use of foraging racks and shavings as enrichment tools for groups of rhesus monkeys (*Macaca mulatta*). *Zoo Biology* **14**, 463–74.

Lyons, J., Young, R. J. & Deag, J. M. (1997) The effects of physical characteristics of the environment and feeding regime on the behavior of captive felids. *Zoo Biology* **16**, 71–83.

McCay, C. M., Maynard, L. A., Sperling, G. & Barnes, L. L. (1939) Retarded growth, life span, ultimate body size, and age changes in the albino rat after feeding diets restricted in calories. *Journal of Nutrition* **18**, 1–13.

McComb, K., Packer, C. & Pusey, A. (1994) Roaring and numerical assessment in contests between groups of female lions, *Panthera leo*. *Animal Behaviour* **47**, 379–87.

McCune, S. (1997) Enriching the environment of the laboratory cat – a review. In: *Proceedings of the Second International Conference on Environmental Enrichment* (ed. B. Holst), pp. 103–17. Copenhagen Zoo, Copenhagen.

McGlone, J. J. (2001) Farm animal welfare in the context of other society issues: toward sustainable systems. *Livestock Production Science* **72**, 75–81.

McGreevy, P. & Nicol, C. (1998) Physiological and behavioral consequences associated with short-term prevention of crib-biting in horses. *Physiology & Behavior* **65**, 15–23.

McGregor, P. K. & Ayling, S. J. (1990) Varied cages results in more aggression in male CFLP mice. *Applied Animal Behaviour Science* **26**, 277–81.

McInerney, J. (1991) A socio-economic perspective on animal-welfare. *Outlook on Agriculture* **20**, 51–6.

McKenzie, S. M., Chamove, A. S. & Feistner, A. T. C. (1986) Floor-coverings and hanging screens alter arboreal monkey behavior. *Zoo Biology* **5**, 339–48.

McLean, J. A., Savory, C. J. & Sparks, N. H. C. (2002) Welfare of male and female broiler chickens in relation to stocking density, as indicated by performance, health and behaviour. *Animal Welfare* **11**, 55–73.

MacPhail, E. M. & Bolhuis, J. J. (2001) The evolution of intelligence: adaptive specializations versus general process. *Biological Reviews* **76**, 341–64.

Maddocks, S. A., Cuthill, I. C., Goldsmith, A. R. & Sherwin, C. M. (2001) Behavioural and physiological effects of absence of ultraviolet wavelengths for domestic chicks. *Animal Behaviour* **62**, 1013–19.

Manning, A. & Dawkins, M. S. (1996) *An Introduction to Animal Behaviour*. Cambridge University Press, Cambridge.

Manosevitz, M. & Joel, U. (1973) Behavioral effects of environmental enrichment in randomly bred mice. *Journal of Comparative and Physiological Psychology* **85**, 373–82.

Manosevitz, M. & Pryor, J. P. (1975) Cage size as a factor in environmental enrichment. *Journal of Comparative and Physiological Psychology* **89**, 648–54.

Manser, M. B. (1999) Response of foraging group members to sentinel calls in suricates, *Suricata suricatta*. *Proceedings of the Royal Society of London Series* B: *Biological Sciences* **266**, 1013–19.

Manteca, X. & Deag, J. M. (1993) Social roles in cattle – a plea for interchange of ideas between primatologists and applied ethnologists. *Animal Welfare* **2**, 339–46.

Maple, T. L. & Findlay, T. W. (1989) Post-occupancy evaluation in the zoo. *Applied Animal Behaviour Science* **18**, 5–18.

Maple, T. L. & Perkin, L. A. (1996) Enclosure furnishings and structural environmental enrichment. In: *Wild Mammals in Captivity* (eds D. G. Kleiman, M. E. Allen, K. V. Thompson, S. Lumpkin & H. Harris), pp. 212–22. University of Chicago Press, Chicago.

Maples, E. G., Haraway, M. M. & Collie, L. (1988) Interactive singing of a male Mueller gibbon with a simulated neighbor. *Zoo Biology*, **7**, 115–22.

Markowitz, H. (1982) *Behavioral Engineering in the Zoo.* Van Nostrand Reinhold, New York.

Markowitz, H., Aday, C. & Gavazzi, A. (1995) Effectiveness of acoustic prey – environmental enrichment for a captive African leopard (*Panthera pardus*). *Zoo Biology* **14**, 371–9.

Markus, N. & Croft, D. B. (1995) Play-behavior and its effects on social-development of common chimpanzees (*Pan troglodytes*). *Primates* **36**, 213–25.

Martin, P. & Bateson, P. (1993) *Measuring Behaviour.* Cambridge University Press, Cambridge.

Martrenchar, A., Huonnic, D. & Cotte, J. P. (2001) Influence of environmental enrichment on injurious pecking and perching behaviour in young turkeys. *British Poultry Science* **42**, 161–70.

Masataka, N. (1993) Effects of experience with live insects on the development of snake fear in squirrel monkeys, *Saimiri sciureus*. *Animal Behaviour* **46**, 741–6.

Masefield, W. (1999) Forage preferences and enrichment in a group of captive Livingstone's fruit bats, *Pteropus livingstonii*. *Dodo – Journal of the Wildlife Preservation Trusts* **35**, 48–56.

Mason, G. & Mendl, M. (1997) Do the stereotypies of pigs, chickens and mink reflect adaptive species differences in the control of foraging? *Applied Animal Behaviour Science* **53**, 45–58.

Mason, G. J. (1991) Stereotypies: a critical review. *Animal Behaviour*, **41**, 1015–37.

Mason, G. J., Cooper, J. & Clarebrough, C. (2001) Frustrations of fur-farmed mink – mink may thrive in captivity but they miss having water to romp about in. *Nature* **410**, 35–6.

Mason, G., McFarland, D. & Garner, J. (1998) A demanding task: using economic techniques to assess animal priorities. *Animal Behaviour* **55**, 1071–5.

Mason, W. A. & Capitanio, J. P. (1988) Formation and expression of filial attachment in rhesus monkeys raised with living and inanimate substitutes. *Developmental Psychobiology* **21**, 401–30.

Matfield, M. (1995) The public debate about animal experimentation. *Atla-Alternatives to Laboratory Animals* **23**, 312–16.

Mather, J. A. (1995) Cognition in cephalopods. *Advances in the Study of Behavior* **24**, 317–53.

Matthews, L. R. & Ladewig, J. (1994) Environmental requirements of pigs measured by behavioural demand functions. *Animal Behaviour* **47**, 713–19.

Matthews, L. R. (1996) Animal welfare and sustainability of production under extensive conditions: a non-EU perspective. *Applied Animal Behaviour Science* **49**, 41–6.

Mellen, J. D. (1991) Factors influencing reproductive success in small exotic felids (*Felis* spp.): a multiple regression analysis. *Zoo Biology* **10**, 95–110.

Mellen, J. D. (1994) Survey and interzoo studies used to address husbandry problems in some zoo vertebrates. *Zoo Biology* **13**, 459–70.

Mellen, J. D. & Ellis, S. (1996) Animal learning and husbandry training. In: *Wild Mammals in Captivity* (eds D. G. Kleiman, M. E. Allen, K. V. Thompson, S. Lumpkin & H. Harris), pp. 88–99. University of Chicago Press, Chicago.

Mellen, J. D., Hayes, M. P. & Shepherdson, D. J. (1998) Captive environments for small felids. In: *Second Nature* (eds D. J. Shepherdson, J. D. Mellen & M. Hutchins), pp. 184–201. Smithsonian Institution Press, Washington.

Mench, J. (1998) Environmental enrichment and the importance of exploratory behaviour. In: *Second Nature* (eds D. J. Shepherdson, J. D. Mellen & M. Hutchins), pp. 30–46. Smithsonian Institution Press, Washington.

Mendl, M. & Newman, H. A. (1997) Social conditions. In: *Animal Welfare* (eds M. C. Appleby & B. O. Hughes), pp. 191–203. CAB International, Cambridge.

Meredith, A. (2002) Chipmunks. In: *BSAVA Manual of Exotic Pets* (eds A. Meredith & S. Redrobe), BSAVA, Gloucester.

Meyer, H. (2000) The rational reason in the German law of animal welfare, regarding the breed and the use of horses. *Pferdeheilkunde* **16**, 229–42.

Meyer-Holzapfel, M. (1968) Abnormal behaviour in zoo animals. In: *Abnormal Behaviour in Animals* (ed. M. W. Fox), pp. 476–503. Saunders, London.

Miller, B., Biggins, D., Vargas, A. *et al.* (1998) The captive environment and reintroduction: the blackfooted ferret as a case study with comments on other taxa. In: *Second Nature* (eds D. J. Shepherdson, J. D. Mellen & M. Hutchins), pp. 97–112. Smithsonian Institution Press, Washington.

Milligan, S. R., Sales, G. D. & Khirnykh, K. (1993) Sound levels in rooms housing laboratory animals – an uncontrolled daily variable. *Physiology & Behavior* **53**, 1067–76.

Mills, A. D. & Faure, J. M. (2000) Ease of capture in lines of Japanese quail (*Coturnix japonica*) subjected to contrasting selection for fear or sociability. *Applied Animal Behaviour Science* **69**, 125–34.

Mills, D. S., Eckley, S. & Cooper, J. J. (2000) Thoroughbred bedding preferences, associated behaviour differences and their implications for equine welfare. *Animal Science* **70**, 95–106.

Mineka, S., Gunnar, M. R. & Champoux, M. (1986) Control and early socio-emotional development: infant rhesus monkeys reared in controllable versus uncontrollable environments. *Child Development* **57**, 1241–56.

Mitchell, D., Becnel, J. R. & Blue, T. (1981) The neophobia-optimality explanation of contrafreeloading rats – a reassessment. *Behavioral and Neural Biology* **32**, 454–62.

Mitchell, G., Herring, F., Obradovich, S. *et al.* (1991) Effects of visitors and cage changes on the behaviors of mangabeys. *Zoo Biology* **10**, 417–23.

Mitchell, G., Tromborg, C. T., Kaufman, J., Bargabus, S., Simoni, R. & Geissler, V. (1992) More on the influence of zoo visitors on the behavior of captive primates. *Applied Animal Behaviour Science* **35**, 189–98.

Moinard, C., Lewis, P. D., Perry, G. C. & Sherwin, C. M. (2001) The effects of light intensity and light source on injuries due to pecking of male domestic turkeys (*Meleagris gallopavo*). *Animal Welfare* **10**, 131–9.

deMonte, M. & LePape, G. (1997) Behavioural effects of cage enrichment in single-caged adult cats. *Animal Welfare* **6**, 53–66.

Moran, G. (1984) Vigilance behavior and alarm calls in a captive group of meerkats, *Suricata suricatta*. *Zeitschrift für Tierpsychologie – Journal of Comparative Ethology* **65**, 228–40.

Moritz, J. (2000) Pet markets: permit and surveillance. *Deutsche Tierarztliche Wochenschrift* **107**, 109–12.

Morris, D. (1964) The response of animals to a restricted environment. *Symposium of the Zoological Society of London* **13**, 99–118.

Morris, P. H., Reddy, V. & Bunting, R. C. (1995) The survival of the cutest: who's responsible for the evolution of the teddy bear? *Animal Behaviour* **50**, 1697–700.

Motl, R. W., Berger, B. G. & Leuschen, P. S. (2000) The role of enjoyment in the exercise-mood relationship. *International Journal of Sport Psychology* **31**, 347–63.

Naka, F., Shiga, T., Yaguchi, M. & Kado, N. (2002) An enriched environment increases noradrenaline concentration in the mouse brain. *Brain Research* **924**, 124–6.

Narjisse, H., Malechek, J. C. & Olsen, J. D. (1997) Influence of odor and taste of monoterpenoids on food selection by anosmic and intact sheep and goats. *Small Ruminant Research*, **23**, 109–15.

Neville, P. (1993) *Pet Sex: The Rude Facts of Life for the Family Dog, Cat and Rabbit*. Sidgwick & Jackson, London.

Nevison, C. M., Hurst, J. L. & Barnard, C. J. (1999) Strain-specific effects of cage enrichment in male laboratory mice (*Mus musculus*). *Animal Welfare* **8**, 361–79.

Newberry, R. C. (1995) Environmental enrichment – increasing the biological relevance of captive environments. *Applied Animal Behaviour Science* **44**, 229–43.

Ng, Y. K. (1995) Towards welfare biology – evolutionary economics of animal consciousness and suffering. *Biology & Philosophy* **10**, 255–85.

Nicol, C. J. (1992) Effects of environmental enrichment and gentle handling on behaviour and fear responses of transported broilers. *Applied Animal Behaviour Science* **33**, 367–80.

Nijman, V. & Heuts, B. A. (2000) Effect of environmental enrichment upon resource holding power in fish in prior residence situations. *Behavioural Processes* **49**, 77–83.

Nilsson, C. (1992) Walking and laying surfaces in livestock houses. In: *Farm Animals and the Environment* (eds C. J. C. Philips & D. Piggins), pp. 93–110. CAB International, Wallingford, Oxford.

Nimon, A. J., Schroter, R. C. & Oxenham, R. K. C. (1996) Artificial eggs: measuring heart rate and effects of disturbance in nesting penguins. *Physiology & Behavior* **60**, 1019–22.

Norgaardnielsen, G., Vestergaard, K. & Simonsen, H. B. (1993) Effects of rearing experience and stimulus enrichment on feather damage in laying hens. *Applied Animal Behaviour Science* 38, 345–52.

Norton, B. C., Hutchins, M., Stevens, E. F. & Maple, T. L. (1995) *Ethics on the Ark*. Smithsonian Institution Press, Washington.

Novak, M. A., Kinsey, J. H., Jorgensen, M. J. & Hazen, T. J. (1998) Effects of puzzle feeders on pathological behavior in individually housed rhesus monkeys. *American Journal of Primatology* 46, 213–27.

Nowak, D. (1993) Problems of animal-welfare during official veterinary surveillance of pet shops. *Deutsche Tierarztliche Wochenschrift* 100, 76–8.

O'Neill, P. L., Novak, M. A. & Suomi, S. J. (1991) Normalizing laboratory-reared rhesus macaque (*Macaca mulatta*) behavior with exposure to complex outdoor enclosures. *Zoo Biology* 10, 237–45.

O'Connell, N. E. & Beattie, V. E. (1999) Influence of environmental enrichment on aggressive behaviour and dominance relationships in growing pigs. *Animal Welfare* 8, 269–79.

O'Connor, K. I. (2000) Mealworm dispensers as environmental enrichment for captive Rodrigues fruit bats (*Pteropus rodricensis*). *Animal Welfare* 9, 123–37.

O'Corry-Crowe, G. M., Suydam, R. S., Rosenberg, A., Frost, K. J. & Dizon, A. E. (1997) Phylogeography, population structure and dispersal patterns of the beluga whale, *Delphinapterus leucas*, in the western Nearctic revealed by mitochondrial DNA. *Molecular Ecology* 6, 955–70.

Odberg, F. O. (1996) Animal welfare science, public discussion and political decisions. *Acta Agriculturae Scandinavica Section a – Animal Science*, 97–103.

Ogden, J. J., Lindburg, D. G. & Maple, T. L. (1993) Preference for structural environmental features in captive lowland gorillas (*Gorilla gorilla gorilla*). *Zoo Biology* 12, 381–95.

Ogden, J. J., Lindburg, D. G. & Maple, T. L. (1994) A preliminary-study of the effects of ecologically relevant sounds on the behavior of captive lowland gorillas. *Applied Animal Behaviour Science* 39, 163–76.

Oldigs, B., Jarfe, A., Baulain, U. & Kallweit, E. (1995a) Investigation on outdoor piglet production in respect to animal-welfare. 2: Evaluation by behavioral traits. *Zuchtungskunde* 67, 288–304.

Oldigs, B., Link, M., Baulain, U. & Kallweit, E. (1995b) Investigation on outdoor piglet production in respect to animal-welfare – 1st Communication – evaluation by performance, technopathies, and physiological reactions. *Zuchtungskunde* 67, 230–44.

Olsen, A. W., Vestergaard, E. M. & Dybkjaer, L. (2000) Roughage as additional rooting substrates for pigs. *Animal Science* 70, 451–6.

Olsson, T., Mohammed, A. K., Donaldson, L. F. & Seckl, J. R. (1995) Transcription factor Ap-2 gene-expression in adult-rat hippocampal regions – effects of environmental manipulations. *Neuroscience Letters* 189, 113–16.

Orgeldinger, M. (1997) Protective and territorial behavior in captive siamangs (*Hylobates syndactylus*). *Zoo Biology* 16, 309–25.

Orlans, F. B. (1996) The three Rs in research and education: a long road ahead in the United States. *Atla-Alternatives to Laboratory Animals* 24, 151–8.

Overall, K. L., Dunham, A. E. & Frank, D. (2001) Frequency of nonspecific clinical signs in dogs with separation anxiety, thunderstorm phobia, and noise phobia, alone or in combination. *Journal of the American Veterinary Medical Association* **219**, 467–73.

Oweis, P. & Spinks, W. L. (2001) Psychological outcomes of physical activity, a theoretical perspective. *Journal of Human Movement* **40**, 351–75.

Pare, W. P. & Kluczynski, J. (1997) Developmental factors modify stress ulcer incidence in a stress-susceptible rat strain. *Journal of Physiology-Paris* **91**, 105–11.

Passariello, P. (1999) Me and my totem: cross-cultural attitudes towards animals. In: *Attitudes to Animals* (ed. F. Dolins), pp. 12–25. Cambridge University Press, Cambridge.

Passig, C., PintoHamuy, T., Moreno, J. P., Rodriguez, C., Rojas, C. & Rosas, R. (1996) Persistence of the cognitive effects of an early stimulation animal model. *Revista Medica de Chile* **124**, 409–16.

Passineau, M. J., Green, E. J. & Dietrich, W. D. (2001) Therapeutic effects of environmental enrichment on cognitive function and tissue integrity following severe traumatic brain injury in rats. *Experimental Neurology* **168**, 373–84.

Patton, M. L., White, A. M., Swaisgood, R. R. *et al.* (2001) Aggression control in a bachelor herd of fringe-eared oryx (*Oryx gazella callotis*), with melengestrol acetate: behavioral and endocrine observations. *Zoo Biology* **20**, 375–88.

Pawlowski, B., Lowen, C. B. & Dunbar, R. I. M. (1998) Neocortex size, social skills and mating success in primates. *Behaviour* **135**, 357–68.

Pedersen, V. (1996) Combined behavioural and physiological measurements as a basis of the assessment of animal welfare. *Acta Agriculturae Scandinavica* Section a – Animal Science, 69–75.

Pedersen, V., Barnett, J. L., Hemsworth, P. H., Newman, E. A. & Schirmer, B. (1998) The effects of handling on behavioural and physiological responses to housing in tether-stalls among pregnant pigs. *Animal Welfare* **7**, 137–50.

Pellew, R. A. (1984) Feeding ecology of a selective browser, the giraffe (*Giraffa camelopardalis tippelskirchi*). *Journal of Zoology* **202**, 57–81.

Pepperberg, I. M. (1983) Cognition in the African grey parrot – preliminary evidence for auditory vocal comprehension of the class concept. *Animal Learning & Behavior* **11**, 179–85.

Pepperberg, I. M. (1993a) Communication between humans and birds, a case-study on the cognitive capabilities of an African gray parrot. *Zeitschrift für Semiotik* **15**, 41–67.

Pepperberg, I. M. (1993b) A review of the effects of social-interaction on vocal learning in African grey parrots (*Psittacus erithacus*). *Netherlands Journal of Zoology* **43**, 104–24.

Pepperberg, I. M. (1994) Numerical competence in an African gray parrots (*Psittacus erithacus*). *Journal of Comparative Psychology* **108**, 36–44.

Pepperberg, I. M. (1998) Out of the mouths of babes . . . and beaks of birds? A broader interpretation of the frame/content theory for the evolution of speech production. *Behavioral and Brain Sciences* **21**, 526–7.

Pepperberg, I. M. & Funk, M. S. (1990) Object permanence in 4 species of psittacine birds – an African gray parrot (*Psittacus erithacus*), an illiger mini macaw (*Ara maracana*), a parakeet (*Melopsittacus undulatus*), and a cockatiel (*Nymphicus hollandicus*). *Animal Learning & Behavior* **18**, 97–108.

Pepperberg, I. M., Sandefer, R. M. & Noel, D. A. (2000) Vocal learning in the grey parrot (*Psittacus erithacus*): effects of species identity and number of trainers. *Journal of Comparative Psychology* **114**, 371–80.

Petit, O. & Thierry, B. (1994) Aggresssion and peaceful interventions in conflicts in tonkean macaques. *Animal Behaviour* **48**, 1427–36.

Pettifer, H. L. (1981) The experimental release of cheetahs (*Acinonyx jubatus*) into a natural environment. In: *Worldwide Furbearer Conference Proceedings* (eds J. A. Chapman & D. Pursley), pp. 1001–24. R. R. Donnelly, Vancouver.

Pham, T. M., Ickes, B., Albeck, D., Soderstrom, S., Granholm, A. C. & Mohammed, A. H. (1999a) Changes in brain nerve growth factor levels and nerve growth factor receptors in rats exposed to environmental enrichment for one year. *Neuroscience* **94**, 279–86.

Pham, T. M., Soderstrom, S., Winblad, B. & Mohammed, A. H. (1999b) Effects of environmental enrichment on cognitive function and hippocampal NGF in the non-handled rats. *Behavioural Brain Research* **103**, 63–70.

Pickering, S., Creighton, E. & Stevenswood, B. (1992) Flock size and breeding success in flamingos. *Zoo Biology* **11**, 229–34.

Pinaud, R., Penner, M. R., Robertson, H. A. & Currie, R. W. (2001) Upregulation of the immediate early gene arc in the brains of rats exposed to environmental enrichment: implications for molecular plasticity. *Molecular Brain Research* **91**, 50–6.

Plaisted, K. C. & Mackintosh, N. J. (1995) Visual-search for cryptic stimuli in pigeons – implications for the search image and search rate hypotheses. *Animal Behaviour* **50**, 1219–32.

Platt, D. M. & Novak, M. A. (1997) Videostimulation as enrichment for captive rhesus monkeys (*Macaca mulatta*). *Applied Animal Behaviour Science* **52**, 139–55.

Pocard, M. (1999) Origin of animal experimentation legislation in the 19th century. *Annales de Chirurgie* **53**, 627–31.

Podberscek, A. L. (1997) Illuminating issues of companion animal welfare through research into human-animal interactions. *Animal Welfare* **6**, 365–72.

Pond, C. M. (1994) Human factors in evolution. In: *Evolution* (ed. P. Skelton), pp. 917–94. The Open University Press, Bath.

Poole, T. (1997) Happy animals make good science. *Laboratory Animals* **31**, 116–24.

Poole, T. B. (1987) Social-behavior of a group of orangutans (*Pongo pygmaeus*) on an artificial island in Singapore Zoological Gardens. *Zoo Biology* **6**, 315–30.

Poole, T. B. (1992) The nature and evolution of behavioural needs in mammals. *Animal Welfare* **1**, 315–30.

Poole, T. B. (1998) Meeting a mammal's psychological needs. In: *Second Nature* (eds D. J. Shepherdson, J. D. Mellen & M. Hutchins), pp. 83–94. Smithsonian Institution Press, Washington.

Poole, T. B. (1999) *UFAW Handbook on the Care and Management of Laboratory Animals.* Blackwell Science, Oxford.

Porsolt, R. D., Roux, S. & Wettstein, J. G. (1995) Animal-models of dementia. *Drug Development Research* **35**, 214–29.

Price, E. & McGrew, W. C. (1990) Cotton-top tamarins in a semi-naturalistic colony. *American Journal of Primatology* **20**, 1–12.

Provenza, F. D. (1995) Postingestive feedback as an elementary determinant of food preference and intake in ruminants. *Journal of Range Management* **48**, 2–17.

Provenza, F. D. (1996) Acquired aversions as the basis for varied diets of ruminants foraging on rangelands. *Journal of Animal Science* **74**, 2010–20.

Provenza, F. D., Lynch, J. J. & Nolan, J. V. (1994) Food aversion conditioned in anesthetized sheep. *Physiology & Behavior* **55**, 429–32.

Prusky, G. T., Reidel, C. & Douglas, R. M. (2000) Environmental enrichment from birth enhances visual acuity but not place learning in mice. *Behavioural Brain Research* **114**, 11–15.

Pryor, K. (1985) *Don't Shoot the Dog*. Bantham Books, New York.

Puppe, B., Schon, P. C. & Wendland, K. (1999) Monitoring of piglets' open field activity and choice behaviour during the replay of maternal vocalization: a comparison between observer and PID technique. *Laboratory Animals* **33**, 215–20.

Rainbird, A. L. (1988) Feeding throughout life. In: *The Waltham Book of Cat and Dog Nutrition* (ed. A. T. B. Edney), pp. 75–96. Pergamon Press, Oxford.

Rasmuson, S., Olsson, T., Henriksson, B. G. *et al.* (1998) Environmental enrichment selectively increases 5-HT1A receptor mRNA expression and binding in the rat hippocampus. *Molecular Brain Research* **53**, 285–90.

Rauw, W. M., Kanis, E., Noordhuizen-Stassen, E. N. & Grommers, F. J. (1998) Undesirable side effects of selection for high production efficiency in farm animals: a review. *Livestock Production Science* **56**, 15–33.

Reade, L. S. & Waran, N. K. (1996) The modern zoo: how do people perceive zoo animals? *Applied Animal Behaviour Science* **47**, 109–18.

Reed, H. J., Wilkins, L. J., Austin, S. D. & Gregory, N. G. (1993) The effect of environmental enrichment during rearing on fear reactions and depopulation trauma in adult caged hens. *Applied Animal Behaviour Science* **36**, 39–46.

Regan, T. (1984) *The Case for Animal Rights*. Routledge, London.

Reinhardt, V. (1989) Behavioral-responses of unrelated adult male rhesus-monkeys familiarized and paired for the purpose of environmental enrichment. *American Journal of Primatology* **17**, 243–8.

Reinhardt, V. (1991) Group formation of previously single-caged adult rhesus macaques for the purpose of environmental enrichment. *Journal of Experimental Animal Science* **34**, 110–15.

Reinhardt, V. (1994) Pair-housing rather than single-housing for laboratory rhesus macaques. *Journal of Medical Primatology* **23**, 426–31.

Reinhardt, V. & Reinhardt, A. (2000) Social enhancement for adult nonhuman primates in research laboratories: a review. *Lab Animal* **29**, 34–41.

Reinhardt, V. & Reinhardt, A. (2002) Housing of laboratory primates. *Animal Welfare* **11**, p. 139.

Reinhardt, V. & Roberts, A. (1997) Effective feeding enrichment for non-human primates: a brief review. *Animal Welfare* **6**, 265–72.

Reinhardt, V., Houser, D., Eisele, S., Cowley, D. & Vertein, R. (1988) Behavioral-responses of unrelated rhesus-monkey females paired for the purpose of environmental enrichment. *American Journal of Primatology* **14**, 135–40.

Rice, T. R., Harvey, H., Kayheart, R. & Torres, C. (1999) Effective strategy for evaluating tactile enrichment devices for singly caged macaques. *Contemporary Topics in Laboratory Animal Science* **38**, 24–6.

Richards, A. F. (1985) *Primates in Nature.* W. H. Freeman and Company, New York.

van Rijzingen, I. M. S., Gispen, W. H. & Spruijt, B. M. (1997) Postoperative environment enrichment attenuates fimbria-fornix lesion-induced impairments in Morris maze performance. *Neurobiology of Learning and Memory* **67**, 21–8.

Roberts, R. L., Roytburd, L. A. & Newman, J. D. (1999) Puzzle feeders and gum feeders as environmental enrichment for common marmosets. *Contemporary Topics in Laboratory Animal Science* **38**, 27–31.

Rooney, N. J. & Bradshaw, J. W. S. (2002) An experimental study of the effects of play upon the dog-human relationships. *Applied Animal Behaviour Science* **75**, 161–76.

Rooney, N. J., Bradshaw, J. W. S. & Robinson, I. H. (2000) A comparison of dog–dog and dog–human play behaviour. *Applied Animal Behaviour Science* **66**, 235–48.

Rosenthal, M. A. & Xanten, W. A. (1996) Structural and keeper considerations in exhibit design. In: *Wild Mammals in Captivity* (eds D. G. Kleiman, M. E. Allen, K. V. Thompson, S. Lumpkin & H. Harris), pp. 212–22. University of Chicago Press, Chicago.

Rosenthal, R. (1979) The 'file drawer problem' and tolerance for null results. *Psychological Bulletin* **86**, 638–41.

Rowan, A. N. & Beck, A. M. (1994) The health benefits of human–animal interactions. *Anthrozoos* **7**, 85–9.

Rowden, J. (2001) Behavior of captive Bulwer's wattled pheasants, *Lophura bulweri* (Galliformes: phasianidae). *Zoo Biology* **20**, 15–25.

Roy, V., Belzung, C., Delarue, C. & Chapillon, P. (2001) Environmental enrichment in BALB/c mice – effects in classical tests of anxiety and exposure to a predatory odor. *Physiology & Behavior* **74**, 313–20.

Rubin, E. S. & Michelson, K. J. (1994) Nursing behavior in dam-reared Russian saiga (*Saiga tatarica tatarica*) at the San Diego Wild Animal Park. *Zoo Biology* **13**, 309–14.

Rumbaugh, D. M., Washburn, D. A. & Savagerumbaugh, S. (1989) On the care of captive chimpanzees: methods of enrichment. In: *Housing, Care and Psychological Wellbeing of Captive and Laboratory Primates* (ed. E. F. Segal), pp. 357–75. Noyes Publications, New Jersey.

Russell, W. M. S. (1995) The development of the 3 Rs concept. *Atla-Alternatives to Laboratory Animals* **23**, 298–304.

Ryder, R. (1989) *Animal Revolution, Changing Attitudes towards Speciesism.* Blackwell Science, Oxford.

Saibaba, P., Sales, G. D., Stodulski, G. & Hau, J. (1996) Behaviour of rats in their home cages: daytime variations and effects of routine husbandry procedures analysed by time sampling techniques. *Laboratory Animals* 30, 13–21.

Sales, G. D., Milligan, S. R. & Khirnykh, K. (1999) Sources of sound in the laboratory animal environment: a survey of the sounds produced by procedures and equipment. *Animal Welfare* 8, 97–115.

Salmon, P. (2001) Effects of physical exercise on anxiety, depression, and sensitivity to stress: a unifying theory. *Clinical Psychology Review*, 21, 33–61.

Sambrook, T. D. & Buchanar-Smith, H. M. (1997) Control and complexity in novel object enrichment. *Animal Welfare* 6, 207–16.

Sandøe, P., Crisp, R. & Holtug, N. (1997) Ethics. In: *Animal Welfare* (eds M. C. Appleby & B. O. Hughes), pp. 3–17. CAB International, Wallingford, Oxford.

Saudargas, R. A. & Drummer, L. C. (1996) Single subject (small N) research designs and zoo research. *Zoo Biology* 15, 173–81.

Schaffer, D., Marquardt, V., Marx, G. & von Borell, E. (2001) Noise in animal housing – a review with emphasis on pig housing. *Deutsche Tierarztliche Wochenschrift* 108, 60–6.

Schapiro, S. J. & Kessel, A. L. (1993) Weight gain among juvenile rhesus macaques – a comparison of enriched and control-groups. *Laboratory Animal Science* 43, 315–18.

Schapiro, S. J., Bloomsmith, M. A., Kessel, A. L. & Shively, C. A. (1993) Effects of enrichment and housing on cortisol response in juvenile rhesus-monkeys. *Applied Animal Behaviour Science* 37, 251–63.

Schapiro, S. J., Porter, L. M., Suarez, S. A. & Bloomsmith, M. A. (1995) The behavior of singly-caged, yearling rhesus-monkeys is affected by the environment outside of the cage. *Applied Animal Behaviour Science* 45, 151–63.

Schapiro, S. J., Bloomsmith, M. A., Suarez, S. A. & Porter, L. M. (1996) Effects of social and inanimate enrichment on the behavior of yearling rhesus monkeys. *American Journal of Primatology* 40, 247–60.

Schapiro, S. J., Nehete, P. N., Perlman, J. E. & Sastry, K. J. (2000) A comparison of cell-mediated immune responses in rhesus macaques housed singly, in pairs, or in groups. *Applied Animal Behaviour Science* 68, 67–84.

Schmidt-Nielsen, K. (1985) *Animal Physiology*. Cambridge University Press, Cambridge.

Schmitz, J. (1994) Requirements for enhanced stimulating conditions in animal housing. *Tierarztliche Umschau* 49, 545–8.

Schrott, L. M., Denenberg, V. H., Sherman, G. F., Waters, N. S., Rosen, G. D. & Galaburda, A. M. (1992) Environmental enrichment, neocortical ectopias, and behavior in the autoimmune Nzb mouse. *Developmental Brain Research* 67, 85–93.

Schuett, G. W. (1996) Fighting dynamics of male copperheads, *Agkistrodon contortrix* (Serpentes, Viperidae): stress-induced inhibition of sexual behavior in losers. *Zoo Biology* 15, 209–21.

Schuppli, C. A. & Fraser, D. (2000) A framework for assessing the suitability of different species as companion animals. *Animal Welfare* 9, 359–72.

Schwitzer, C. & Kaumanns, W. (2001) Body weights of ruffed lemurs (*Varecia variegata*) in European zoos with reference to the problem of obesity. *Zoo Biology* 20, 261–9.

Scott, P. W., Stevenson, M. F., Cooper, J. E. & Cooper, M. E. (2000) *Secretary of State's Standards of Modern Zoo Practice*. Her Majesty's Stationery Office, Norwich.

Seidensticker, J. & Doherty, J. G. (1996) Integrating animal behavior and exhibit design. In: *Wild Mammals in Captivity* (eds D. G. Kleiman, M. E. Allen, K. V. Thompson, S. Lumpkin & H. Harris), pp. 180–90. University of Chicago Press, Chicago.

Seidensticker, J. & Forthman, D. L. (1998) Evolution, ecology, and enrichment: basic considerations for wild animals in zoos. In: *Second Nature* (eds D. J. Shepherdson, J. D. Mellen & M. Hutchins), pp. 15–29. Smithsonian Institution Press Washington.

Seier, J. V. & deLange, P. W. (1996) A mobile cage facilitates periodic social contact and exercise for singly caged adult vervet monkeys. *Journal of Medical Primatology* 25, 64–8.

Seksel, K. & Lindeman, M. J. (2001) Use of clomipramine in treatment of obsessive-compulsive disorder, separation anxiety and noise phobia in dogs: a preliminary, clinical study. *Australian Veterinary Journal* 79, 252–6.

Seligman, M. E. P. (1975) *Helpessness: On Depression, Development and Death*. W. H. Freeman, San Francisco.

Serpell, J. A. (1996) Evidence for an association between pet behavior and owner attachment levels. *Applied Animal Behaviour Science* 47, 49–60.

Serpell, J. A. (1999) Sheep in wolves' clothing? Attitudes to animals among farmers and scientists. In: *Attitudes to Animals* (ed. F. Dolins), pp. 26–33. Cambridge University Press, Cambridge.

Shepherdson, D. J. (1989) Improving animals lives in captivity through environmental enrichment. In: *Euroniche Conference Proceedings, Edinburgh, Scotland* (eds B. S. Close, F. Dolins & G. J. Mason), pp. 91–102. Humane Education Centre, London.

Shepherdson, D. J. (1994) The role of environmental enrichment in the captive breeding and reintroduction of endangered species. In: *Creative Conservation: Interactive Management of Wild and Captive Animals* (eds G. Mace, P. Olney & A. T. C. Feistner), pp. 167–77. Chapman & Hall, London.

Shepherdson, D. J. (1999) New perspectives on the design and management of captive animal environments. In: *Attitudes to Animals* (ed. F. Dolins), pp. 143–51. Cambridge University Press, Cambridge.

Shepherdson, D. J., Carlstead, K., Mellen, J. D. & Seidensticker, J. (1993) The influence of food presentation on the behavior of small cats in confined environments. *Zoo Biology* 12, 203–16.

Shepherdson, D. J., Mellen, J. D. & Hutchins, M. (1998) *Second Nature*. Smithsonian Institution Press, Washington.

Sherwin, C. M. (1993) Pecking behavior of laying hens provided with a simple motorized environmental enrichment device. *British Poultry Science* 34, 235–40.

Sherwin, C. M. (1998) The use and perceived importance of three resources which provide caged laboratory mice the opportunity for extended locomotion. *Applied Animal Behaviour Science* 55, 353–67.

Sherwin, C. M., Lewis, P. D. & Perry, G. C. (1999a) The effects of environmental enrichment and intermittent lighting on the behaviour and welfare of male domestic turkeys. *Applied Animal Behaviour Science* 62, 319–33.

Sherwin, C. M., Lewis, P. D. & Perry, G. C. (1999b) Effects of environmental enrichment, fluorescent and intermittent lighting on injurious pecking amongst male turkey poults. *British Poultry Science* 40, 592–8.

Shimoji, M., Bowers, C. L. & Crockett, C. M. (1993) Initial response to the introduction of a PVC perch by singly caged *Macaca fascicularis*. *Laboratory Primate Newsletter* **32**, 8–11.

Shomer, N. H., Peikert, S. & Terwilliger, G. (2001) Enrichment-toy trauma in a New Zealand white rabbit. *Contemporary Topics in Laboratory Animal Science* **40**, 31–2.

Simpson, B. S. (2000) Canine separation anxiety. *Compendium on Continuing Education for the Practicing Veterinarian* **22**, 328–38.

Singer, P. (1975) *Animal Liberation*. Jonathan Cape, London.

Smaje, L. H., Smith, J. A., Ewbank, R. *et al.* (1998) Advancing refinement of laboratory animal use. *Laboratory Animals* **32**, 137–42.

Smidt, D., Oldigs, B., Augustin, C. *et al.* (1992) Developments and perspectives in pig farming as related to animal-welfare – status-report of the working group animal-welfare of the Senate of the Federal Ministry of Food, Agriculture and Forestry, Federal Republic of Germany. *Landbauforschung Volkenrode* **42**, 229–46.

Smith, L. K., Field, E. F., Forgie, M. L. & Pellis, S. M. (1996) Dominance and age-related changes in the play fighting of intact and post-weaning castrated male rats (*Rattus norvegicus*). *Aggressive Behavior* **22**, 215–26.

Soffie, M., Hahn, K., Terao, E. & Eclancher, F. (1999) Behavioural and glial changes in old rats following environmental enrichment. *Behavioural Brain Research* **101**, 37–49.

Sommerville, B. A. & Broom, D. M. (1998) Olfactory awareness. *Applied Animal Behaviour Science* **57**, 269–86.

Spijkerman, R. P., Dienske, H., vanHooff, J. A. R. A. M. & Jens, W. (1996) Differences in variability, interactivity and skills in social play of young chimpanzees living in peer groups and in a large family zoo group. *Behaviour* **133**, 717–39.

Spinka, M., Newberry, R. C. & Bekoff, M. (2001) Mammalian play: training for the unexpected. *Quarterly Review of Biology* **76**, 141–68.

Spira, H. (1991) Animal rights and toxicology – a quiet but profound revolution. *Food and Drug Law Journal* **46**, 89–95.

Spring, S. E., Clifford, J. O. & Tomko, D. L. (1997) Effect of environmental enrichment devices on behaviors of single- and group-housed squirrel monkeys (*Saimiri sciureus*). *Contemporary Topics in Laboratory Animal Science* **36**, 72–5.

Staddon, J. E. R. (1987) Operant behavior. In: *The Oxford Companion to Animal Behaviour* (ed. D. McFarland), pp. 426–9. Oxford University Press, Oxford.

Stafford, B. J., Rosenberger, A. L. & Beck, B. B. (1994) Locomotion of free-ranging golden lion tamarins (*Leontopithecus rosalia*) at the National Zoological Park. *Zoo Biology* **13**, 333–44.

Steinigeweg, W. (2000) Keeping of pets – assessment of accessories. *Deutsche Tierärztliche Wochenschrift* **107**, 126–30.

Sterling, E. J. & Povinelli, D. J. (1999) Tool use, aye-ayes, and sensorimotor intelligence. *Folia Primatologica* **70**, 8–16.

Sternglanz, S. H., Gray, J. L. & Murakami, M. (1977) Adult preferences for infantile facial features: an ethological approach. *Animal Behaviour* **25**, 108–15.

Stevens, E. F. (1991) Flamingo breeding – the role of group displays. *Zoo Biology* **11**, 53–63.

Stevens, E. F. & Pickett, C. (1994) Managing the social environments of flamingos for reproductive success. *Zoo Biology* **13**, 501–7.

Stevens, E. F., Beaumont, J. H., Cusson, E. W. & Fowler, J. (1992) Nesting-behavior in a flock of chilean flamingos. *Zoo Biology* **11**, 209–14.

Stevenson, M. F., Dryden, H., Alabaster, A. & Wren, C. (1994) The new penguin enclosure at Edinburgh Zoo: the palace for the 1990s. *International Zoo Yearbook* **33**, 9–15.

Stirling, I. (1990) *Polar Bears*. University of Michigan Press, Ann Arbor.

Stoinski, T. S., Hoff, M. P., Lukas, K. E. & Maple, T. L. (2001) A preliminary behavioral comparison of two captive all-male gorilla groups. *Zoo Biology* **20**, 27–40.

Stolba, A. & Wood-Gush, D. G. M. (1984) The identification of behavioural key features and their incorporation into a housing design for pigs. *Annales de Recherches Vétérinaires* **15**, 287–98.

Stolba, A. & Wood-Gush, D. G. M. (1989) The behaviour of pigs in a semi-natural environment. *Animal Production* **48**, 419–25.

Swaisgood, R. R., White, A. M., Zhou, X. P. *et al.* (2001) A quantitative assessment of the efficacy of an environmental enrichment programme for giant pandas. *Animal Behaviour* **61**, 447–57.

Synder, R. (1977) Putting the wild back into the Zoo. *International Zoo News* **24**, 11–18.

Takeuchi, Y., Houpt, K. A. & Scarlett, J. M. (2000) Evaluation of treatments for separation anxiety in dogs. *Journal of the American Veterinary Medical Association* **217**, 342–5.

Tang, Y. P., Wang, H., Feng, R., Kyin, M. & Tsien, J. Z. (2001) Differential effects of enrichment on learning and memory function in NR2B transgenic mice. *Neuropharmacology* **41**, 779–90.

Tees, R. C. (1999a) The influences of rearing environment and neonatal choline dietary supplementation on spatial learning and memory in adult rats. *Behavioural Brain Research* **105**, 173–88.

Tees, R. C. (1999b) The influences of sex, rearing environment, and neonatal choline dietary supplementation on spatial and nonspatial learning and memory in adult rats. *Developmental Psychobiology* **35**, 328–42.

Terlouw, E. M. C. & Lawrence, A. B. (1993) Long-term effects of food allowance and housing on development of stereotypies in pigs. *Applied Animal Behaviour Science* **38**, 103–26.

Terlouw, E. W. C., Schouten, W. G. P. & Ladewig, J. (1997) Physiology. In: *Animal Welfare* (eds M. C. Appleby & B. O. Hughes), pp. 143–58. CAB International, Wallingford, Oxford.

Terranova, C. J. & Coffman, B. S. (1997) Body weights of wild and captive lemurs. *Zoo Biology* **16**, 17–30.

Thodberg, K., Jensen, K. H., Herskin, M. S. & Jorgensen, E. (1999) Influence of environmental stimuli on nest building and farrowing behaviour in domestic sows. *Applied Animal Behaviour Science* **63**, 131–44.

Thomas, W. D. & Maruska, E. J. (1996) Mixed-species exhibits with mammals. In: *Wild Mammals in Captivity* (eds D. G. Kleiman, M. E. Allen, K. V. Thompson, S. Lumpkin & H. Harris), pp. 204–11. University of Chicago Press, Chicago.

Timmermans, P. J. A., Vochteloo, J. D., Vossen, J. M. H., Roder, E. L. & Duijghuisen, J. A. H. (1994) Persistent neophobic behavior in monkeys – a habit or trait. *Behavioural Processes* **31**, 177–96.

Tinbergen, N. (1951) *The Study of Instinct*. Oxford University Press, Oxford.

Todd, I. C., Wosornu, D., Stewart, I. & Wild, T. (1992) Cardiac rehabilitation following myocardial-infarction – a practical approach. *Sports Medicine* **14**, 243–59.

Torasdotter, M., Metsis, M., Henriksson, B. G., Winblad, B. & Mohammed, A. H. (1996) Expression of neurotrophin-3 mRNA in the rat visual cortex and hippocampus is influenced by environmental conditions. *Neuroscience Letters* **218**, 107–10.

Torasdotter, M., Metsis, M., Henriksson, B. G., Winblad, B. & Mohammed, A. H. (1998) Environmental enrichment results in higher levels of nerve growth factor mRNA in the rat visual cortex and hippocampus. *Behavioural Brain Research* **93**, 83–90.

Tudge, C. (1992) *Last Animals at the Zoo*. Oxford University Press, Oxford.

Turner, D. C. (1997) Treating canine and feline behaviour problems and advising clients. *Applied Animal Behaviour Science* **52**, 199–204.

Van de Weerd, H. A., Baumans, V., Koolhaas, J. M. & van Zutphen, L. F. M. (1994) Strain-specific behavioral-response to environmental enrichment in the mouse. *Journal of Experimental Animal Science* **36**, 117–27.

Van de Weerd, H. A., VanLoo, P. L. P., van Zutphen, L. F. M., Koolhaas, J. M. & Baumans, V. (1997) Nesting material as environmental enrichment has no adverse effects on behavior and physiology of laboratory mice. *Physiology & Behavior* **62**, 1019–28.

VanWaas, M. & Soffie, M. (1996) Differential environmental modulations on locomotor activity, exploration and spatial behaviour in young and old rats. *Physiology & Behavior* **59**, 265–71.

Veasey, J. S. (1993) *An Investigation into the Behaviour of Captive Tigers* (Panthera tigris) *and the Effect of their Enclosure on Behaviour*. BSc thesis, University of London, London.

Veasey, J. S., Waran, N. K. & Young, R. J. (1996a) On comparing the behaviour of zoo housed animals with wild conspecifics as a welfare indicator, using the giraffe (*Giraffa camelopardalis*) as a model. *Animal Welfare* **5**, 139–53.

Veasey, J. S., Waran, N. K. & Young, R. J. (1996b) On comparing the behaviour of zoo housed animals with wild conspecifics as a welfare indicator. *Animal Welfare* **5**, 13–24.

van Veen, T. W. S. (1999) Agricultural policy and sustainable livestock development. *International Journal for Parasitology* **29**, 7–15.

Vick, S. J., Anderson, J. R. & Young, R. (2000) Maracas for *Macaca*? Evaluation of three potential enrichment objects in two species of zoo-housed macaques. *Zoo Biology* **19**, 181–91.

Voith, V. L. & Borchelt, P. L. (1985) Separation anxiety in dogs. *Compendium on Continuing Education for the Practicing Veterinarian* **7**, 42–52.

de Waal, F. B. M. (1983) *Chimpanzee Politics*. Unwin Paperbacks, London.

de Waal, F. B. M. (1989) The myth of a simple relation between space and aggression in captive primates. *Zoo Biology Supplement* **1**, 141–9.

Wainwright, P. E., Levesque, S., Krempulec, L., Bulmanfleming, B. & McCutcheon, D. (1993) Effects of environmental enrichment on cortical depth and Morris-maze performance in B6d2f2 mice exposed prenatally to ethanol. *Neurotoxicology and teratology* **15**, 11–20.

Wainwright, P. E., Huang, Y. S., Bulmanfleming, B., Levesque, S. & McCutcheon, D. (1994) The effects of dietary fatty-acid composition combined with environmental enrichment on brain and behavior in mice. *Behavioural Brain Research* **60**, 125–36.

Waser, P. M. & Brown, C. H. (1984) Is there a sound window for primate communication. *Behavioral Ecology and Sociobiology* **15**, 73–6.

Washburn, D. A., Harper, S. & Rumbaugh, D. M. (1994) Computer-task testing of rhesus-monkeys (*Macaca mulatta*) in the social milieu. *Primates* **35**, 343–51.

Waterhouse, A. (1996) Animal welfare and sustainability of production under extensive conditions – a European perspective. *Applied Animal Behaviour Science* **49**, 29–40.

Webster, A. J. F. (1982) The economics of farm animal-welfare. *International Journal for the Study of Animal Problems* **3**, 301–6.

Webster, A. J. F. (2001) Farm animal welfare: the five freedoms and the free market. *Veterinary Journal* **161**, 229–37.

Wechsler, B. (1991) Stereotypies in Polar Bears. *Zoo Biology* **10**, 177–88.

Wegner, W. (1993) Pet breeding and animal-welfare. *Tierarztliche Umschau* **48**, 213–8.

Weinsier, R. L., Hunter, G. R., Heini, A. F., Goran, M. I. & Sell, S. M. (1998) The etiology of obesity: relative contribution of metabolic factors, diet, and physical activity. *American Journal of Medicine* **105**, 145–50.

Wells, D. L. & Hepper, P. G. (2000a) The influence of environmental change on the behaviour of sheltered dogs. *Applied Animal Behaviour Science* **68**, 151–62.

Wells, D. L. & Hepper, P. G. (2000b) Prevalence of behaviour problems reported by owners of dogs purchased from an animal rescue shelter. *Applied Animal Behaviour Science* **69**, 55–65.

Wemelsfelder, F. (1997) The scientific validity of subjective concepts in models of animal welfare. *Applied Animal Behaviour Science* **53**, 75–88.

Wemelsfelder, F. (2001) The inside and outside aspects of consciousness: complementary approaches to the study of animal emotion. *Animal Welfare* **10**, S129–39.

Wemelsfelder, F. & Birke, L. (1997) Environmental Challenge. In: *Animal Welfare* (eds M. C. Appleby & B. O. Hughes), pp. 35–47. CAB International, Wallingford, Oxford.

Wemelsfelder, F. & Lawrence, A. B. (2001) Qualitative assessment of animal behaviour as an on-farm welfare-monitoring tool. *Acta Agriculturae Scandinavica Section a-Animal Science*, 21–5.

Wemelsfelder, F., Haskell, M., Mendl, M. T., Calvert, S. & Lawrence, A. B. (2000a) Diversity of behaviour during novel object tests is reduced in pigs housed in substrate-impoverished conditions. *Animal Behaviour* **60**, 385–94.

Wemelsfelder, F., Hunter, E. A., Mendl, M. T. & Lawrence, A. B. (2000b) The spontaneoous qualitative assessment of behavioural expressions in pigs: first explorations of a novel methodology for integrative animal welfare measurement. *Applied Animal Behaviour Science* **67**, 193–215.

Wemelsfelder, F., Hunter, T. E. A., Mendl, M. T. & Lawrence, A. B. (2001) Assessing the 'whole animal'. a free choice profiling approach. *Animal Behaviour* **62**, 209–20.

Weyerer, S. & Kupfer, B. (1994) Physical exercise and psychological health. *Sports Medicine* **17**, 108–16.

Wheler, C. L. & Fa, J. E. (1995) Enclosure utilization and activity of Round Island geckos (*Phelsuma guentheri*). *Zoo Biology* **14**, 361–9.

Whitehead, M. (1995) Saying It with genes, species and habitats – biodiversity education and the role of zoos. *Biodiversity and Conservation* **4**, 664–70.

Wiedenmayer, C. (1998) Food hiding and enrichment in captive Asian elephants. *Applied Animal Behaviour Science* **56**, 77–82.

Wiepkema, P. R. (1990) Stress: ethological implications. In: *Psychobiology of Stress* (eds S. Puglisi-Allegra & A. Oliverio), pp. 1–13. Kluwer, Dordrecht.

Williams, B. G., Waran, N. K., Carruthers, J. & Young, R. J. (1996) The effect of a moving bait on the behaviour of captive cheetahs (*Acinonyx jubatus*). *Animal Welfare* **5**, 271–81.

Williams, B. M., Luo, Y., Ward, C., Redd, K., Gibson, R., Kuczaj, S. A. & McCoy, J. G. (2001) Environmental enrichment: effects on spatial memory and hippocampal CREB immunoreactivity. *Physiology & Behavior* **73**, 649–58.

Wilson, L. L., Terosky, T. L., Stull, C. L. & Stricklin, W. R. (1999) Effects of individual housing design and size on behavior and stress indicators of special-fed Holstein veal calves. *Journal of Animal Science* **77**, 1341–7.

Winocur, G. & Greenwood, C. E. (1999) The effects of high fat diets and environmental influences on cognitive performance in rats. *Behavioural Brain Research* **101**, 153–61.

Winskill, L., Waran, N. K., Channing, C. & Young, R. J. (1995) Stereotypies in the stabled horse: causes, treatment and prevention. *Current Science* **69**, 310–6.

Winskill, L. C., Waran, N. K. & Young, R. J. (1996) The effect of a foraging device (a modified 'Edinburgh foodball') on the behaviour of the stabled horse. *Applied Animal Behaviour Science* **48**, 25–35.

Wood, W. (1998) Interactions among environmental enrichment, viewing crowds, and zoo chimpanzees (*Pan troglodytes*). *Zoo Biology* **17**, 211–30.

Woodcock, E. A. & Richardson, R. (2000) Effects of environmental enrichment on rate of contextual processing and discriminative ability in adult rats. *Neurobiology of Learning and Memory* **73**, 1–10.

Wood-Gush, D. G. M. & Vestergaard, K. (1991) The seeking of novelty and its relation to play. *Animal Behaviour* **42**, 599–606.

Wood-Gush, D. G. M. & Vestergaard, K. (1993) Inquisitive exploration in pigs. *Animal Behaviour* **45**, 185–7.

Wormell, D. & Brayshaw, M. (2000) The design and redevelopment of New World primate accommodation at Jersey Zoo: a naturalistic approach. *Dodo – Journal of the Wildlife Preservation Trusts* **36**, 9–19.

Wright, J. & Lashnits, J. W. (1994) *Is Your Cat Crazy? Solutions from the Casebook of a Cat Therapist*. Simon and Shuster, New York.

Wurbel, H., Chapman, R. & Rutland, C. (1998) Effect of feed and environmental enrichment on development of stereotypic wire-gnawing in laboratory mice. *Applied Animal Behaviour Science* **60**, 69–81.

Xerri, C., Coq, J. O., Merzenich, M. M. & Jenkins, W. M. (1996) Experience-induced plasticity of cutaneous maps in the primary somatosensory cortex of adult monkeys and rats. *Journal of Physiology–Paris* **90**, 277–87.

Yerkes, R. M. (1925) *Almost Human.* Century, New York.

Young, D., Lawlor, P. A., Leone, P., Dragunow, M. & During, M. J. (1999) Environmental enrichment inhibits spontaneous apoptosis, prevents seizures and is neuroprotective. *Nature Medicine* **5**, 448–53.

Young, R. J. (1993) Factors affecting foraging motivation in the domestic pig. PhD Thesis, University of Edinburgh, Edinburgh.

Young, R. J. (1997) The importance of food presentation for animal welfare and conservation. *Proceedings of the Nutrition Society* **56**, 1095–104.

Young, R. J. (1998) Behavioural studies of guenons, *Cercopithecus* spp. at Edinburgh Zoo. *International Zoo Yearbook* **36**, 49–56.

Young, R. J. (1999) The behavioural requirements of farm animals for psychological well-being and survival. In: *Attitudes to Animals: Differing Views in Animal Welfare.* (ed. F. Dolins), pp. 77–100. Cambridge University Press, Cambridge.

Young, R. J. & Lawrence, A. B. (1996) The effects of high and low rates of reinforcement on the behaviour of pigs. *Applied Animal Behaviour Science* **49**, 365–74.

Young, R. J., Carruthers, J. & Lawrence, A. B. (1994) The effect of a foraging device (the Edinburgh Foodball) on the behavior of pigs. *Applied Animal Behaviour Science* **39**, 237–47.

Young, R. J., Macleod, H. A. & Lawrence, A. B. (1994a) Effect of manipulation design on operant responding in pigs. *Animal Behaviour* **47**, 1488–90.

Zasloff, R. L. (1996) Measuring attachment to companion animals: a dog is not a cat is not a bird. *Applied Animal Behaviour Science* **47**, 43–8.

Zasloff, R. L. & Hart, L. A. (1998) Attitudes and care practices of cat caretakers in Hawaii. *Anthrozoos* **11**, 242–8.

Zhang, G. Q., Swaisgood, R. R., Wei, R. P. *et al.* (2000) A method for encouraging maternal care in the giant panda. *Zoo Biology* **19**, 53–63.

Zimmermann, A. & Feistner, A. T. C. (1996) Effects of feeding enrichment on ruffed lemurs, *Varecia variegata* and *Varecia v rubra. Dodo – Journal of the Wildlife Preservation Trusts* **32**, 67–75.

Zimmermann, A., Stauffacher, M., Langhans, W. & Wurbel, H. (2001) Enrichment-dependent differences in novelty exploration in rats can be explained by habituation. *Behavioural Brain Research* **121**, 11–20.

van Zutphen, L. F. M. & van der Valk, J. B. F. (2001) Developments on the implementation of the three Rs in research and education. *Toxicology in Vitro* **15**, 591–5.

Glossary

Appetitive behaviour: the expression of goal-seeking behaviour e.g. foraging.

Behavioural conditioning/modification: the changing of animal behaviour by a human care-giver using rewards e.g. operant conditioning.

Behavioural economics: an approach to studying the things that animals want by investigating whether or not they behave like logical human consumers i.e. do they try to maximise cost–benefit ratios in their behavioural expression.

Biological functioning: a definition of animal welfare that refers to the operation of animal biological systems within normal limits.

Care-giver: anyone whose profession is to look after captive animals e.g. zoo keeper.

Cartesian dualism: a rationalist philosophical standpoint proposed by Rene Descartes, that views humans as possessors of a separate body and mind, and animals as only possessing a body, the implication being that animals cannot suffer.

Choice test: the experimental investigation into the preferences of animals for different resources or different kinds of the same resource (often carried out using a 'T'-maze).

Consummatory behaviour: the expression of behaviour once a goal has been found e.g. feeding.

Emotionality: the degree of behavioural reactivity of animals to new or novel situations.

Euthanasia: the humane killing of animals.

Fixed-action patterns: innate and highly stylised behavioural responses of animals to certain stimuli or situations e.g. the putting of food into an open mouth by adult birds.

Free-ranging environments: animals released into an area, such as a zoo, without any apparent barriers or enclosure but with the provision of food and shelter.

Habituation: a form of non-associative learning in which animals initially respond to a neutral stimuli but quickly stop responding when they learn that it has no consequences for them.

Hard architecture: a style of architecture for animal housing that focuses on the needs of hygiene. These enclosures tend to be constructed of concrete and metal and are now considered defunct by many animal welfare scientists due to advances in veterinary medicine.

Hedonistic behaviour: pleasure-seeking behaviour.

Individual variation: the statistical differences between individuals, e.g. weight or behavioural response.

Information gathering: the expression of behaviour (usually exploratory) with the sole objective of collecting information about the environment that may be useful in the future.

Innate behaviours: behaviour patterns that are in place at birth and therefore do not need to be learned. However, these behaviours may be modified by the learning process.

Intensive farming: the rearing of meat animals usually in highly confined conditions e.g. a battery hen housed in a small cage.

K-selected species: species that normally produce few offspring that develop into adults slowly and express parental care e.g. primates.

Learned helplessness: the behaviour arising from a situation where the animal learns that whatever it tries to do to avoid an undesirable situation, it doesn't work. The animal eventually becomes completely unresponsive to the situation and to any stimuli presented to it.

Life-history strategy: the behaviour and physical developmental plan of the animal e.g. the speed of sexual maturation with its associated changes in behaviour and anatomy.

Neocortex ratio: the ratio of the size of the 'thinking' part of the brain (the cortex) to the size of the rest of the brain (the areas that control bodily processes).

Operant behaviour: the expression of a behaviour that is reinforced by the animal obtaining a reward e.g. a hunting lion kills a gazelle.

Reintroduction: the placing of captive-bred animals into a wild environment where they had previously become extinct. Reintroduction is a conservation tool.

R-selected species: species that normally produce offspring in great numbers that develop into adults rapidly and do not express parental care, e.g. fish.

Schedules of reinforcement: the pattern of reward that an animal receives. The reward is often given during training and usually relates to the number of times a particular behaviour is expressed.

Species-specific behaviour: the temporal and physical form of particular behaviour patterns as expressed by one particular species, e.g. the hunting behaviour of cheetahs.

Utilisable space: the amount of space in an environment that the animal wishes to use. This can range from 10–100 % depending on environmental design.

Index

Page numbers in *italics* refer to figures, those in **bold** to tables.